A Spiritual Companion
to Infertility

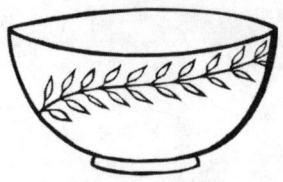

A Spiritual Companion to Infertility

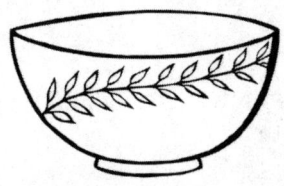

Julie Irwin Zimmerman

PUBLICATIONS

A SPIRITUAL COMPANION TO INFERTILITY
by Julie Irwin Zimmerman

Edited by L.C. Fiore
Cover design by Tom A. Wright
Text design and typesetting by Patricia A. Lynch

Published by ACTA Publications, 5559 W. Howard Street, Skokie, IL 60077, (800) 397-2282, www.actapublications.com.

Library of Congress Number: 2008942231
ISBN: 978-0-87946-389-2
Printed in the United States of America by Versa Press
Year 17 16 15 14 13 12 11 10 09
Printing 10 09 08 07 06 05 04 03 02 First Edition

Contents

Introduction 9

Chapter One – Why, God? 17

Chapter Two – Men, Women and Marriage 35

Chapter Three – The Isolation of Infertility 55

Chapter Four – Loving Ourselves
as God Loves Us 75

Chapter Five – Special Situations
(Miscarriages, Secondary Infertility,
Step-parenting and Infertility) 91

Chapter Six – Making Decisions 105

Chapter Seven – The Morality of Treatment 117

Chapter Eight – Moving On 137

Chapter Nine – Other Options: Adoption 149

Chapter Ten – Other Options:
A Family of Two 165

Chapter Eleven – Waiting in Hope 177

Infertility Resources 189

References 191

To Erik, Oscar and Ingrid —
A family created through
Marriage, birth, adoption,
And most of all, love.

Introduction

To wait open-endedly is an enormously radical attitude toward life. So is to trust that something will happen to us that is far beyond our imaginings. So, too, is giving up control over our future and letting God define our life, trusting that God moulds us according to God's love and not according to our fear. The spiritual life is a life in which we wait, actively present to the moment, trusting that new things will happen to us, new things that are far beyond our own imagination, fantasy, or prediction. That, indeed, is a very radical stance toward life in a world preoccupied with control.

Henri J. M. Nouwen

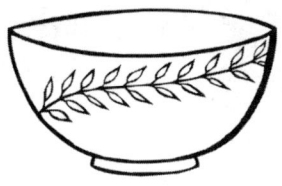

ON MOTHER'S DAY 1998, I sat in church and daydreamed about how joyful the holiday would be for us the following spring. My husband and I, married the previous year, had decided to have a baby. We had been trying for a few months, and I figured we'd conceive soon—just in time to have our newborn with us at church next Mother's Day. Because we were both in our thirties, I knew there was a greater chance that we'd have trouble conceiving. But most of my friends had gotten pregnant without difficulty, and I assumed it would be the same for us. I was full of anticipation and hope as I sat watching the mothers around us tending to their babies.

By Christmas, though, it was clear there was a problem. Nearly a year had passed and still no sign of pregnancy. The months developed an unwelcome rhythm, beginning in hope, proceeding through anxiety, and ending in tears. My prayer life had taken on the same rhythm: first, optimistic appeals for God to grant us a pregnancy, then more frantic pleas for help getting through the month, and finally a silent anguish when I felt my prayers had been ignored once again. We visited our doctor, were referred to specialists, and scoured the Internet for information. Slowly our quest for a child took over our lives.

On Mother's Day 1999, we went to church empty-handed, and I cried through much of the service. The following year was even worse. More than two years had passed, we had spent thousands of dollars trying to conceive, and yet we were no closer to parenthood than when we began. I wondered what we had done to deserve this, why our simple wish for a child had not yet been granted. Was there a lesson in all of this, a reason why we had to suffer for something that seemed to come so easily to everyone else?

The ordeal of infertility is difficult physically. We endure painful shots, embarrassing questions, and more exams than we care to remember. It is difficult financially, as we struggle to pay for expensive drugs and specialists that insurance doesn't cover. It is difficult emotionally and mentally, as months of waiting turn into years, and we put life plans on hold indefinitely.

Are we being punished for something we've done? Can't God hear our desperate pleas?

But for many of us, the most difficult aspect of infertility is how it affects us spiritually. Our God, who feels so near when we begin to plan for a family, suddenly seems absent. Our desperate prayers appear to fall on deaf ears. We beg, plead, bargain, scold—and every month, it feels like wasted effort. We wonder, where is God? Are we being punished for something we've done? Can't God hear our desperate pleas? Why must we suffer like this?

Our other relationships often suffer as well. Our marriage can strain from the pressure, as we face difficult decisions and conflicting priorities. We find it hard to talk to our closest friends and relatives about what we're going through, and even strangers on the street may upset us if they're pregnant or carrying a baby. Our churches sometimes fail to offer the comfort they should. Our self-image suffers as we face guilt, envy, shame and grief.

The sadness we feel as we see our dreams die is as deep as when someone we love dies, but the sadness of infertility returns month after month, often with no end in sight. As with all great suffering, we are changed forever by it. Whether it's been a few months or ten years, whether we end up with a houseful of children or none, adopted or biological, we will always carry the scars of infertility with us. Even now, after giving birth to one child and adopting another, I still can't say that I understand why my husband and I had to endure such difficulty forming our family.

But we must remember—even in those moments when it seems that we may never recover from the pain—that the struggle to have a child presents us with a chance to grow in our faith, to understand God and ourselves better, to strengthen our relationships, and to prepare us for the road ahead. As my husband and I struggled to have a child, we were weighed down by frustration and confusion. But during this time I came to know God better and speak with God more freely— even if that meant speaking in anger sometimes. This particular pain helped me to understand what Jesus did when he willingly accepted his Cross. It taught me patience, deepened my understanding of others' suffering, and prepared me for the day when I finally became a mother.

There is consolation in our faith, and encouragement, even if it's hard to see month after disappointing month. If we allow ourselves the room to do what we need to— whether it's to ask questions, mourn, pray or rage—we may find our way to a deeper, more mature faith: one that understands there are things we will never understand in this life.

We must remember too that the crisis of infertility does not last forever. At some point, everyone finds a way out of this dark place. Some conceive a child; others adopt; still others decide to use their talents and time in different, equally-important ways. And these terrible emotions we feel now—envy and loss, shame and grief— will someday be a distant memory. Someday we'll be able to smile at expectant parents or hold the newborn babies that used to upset us so much when we were suffering. Someday we'll see them as gifts of God's good creation, the same God who will help us resolve our own crisis. No one knows if that someday is just around the corner or a long way off. But be assured that it will come.

PRAYER AND REFLECTION

Psalm 69:13-17

But as for me, my prayer is to you, O Lord, at an acceptable time, O God, in the abundance of your steadfast love, answer me. With your faithful help rescue me from sinking in the mire; let me be delivered from my enemies and from deep waters. Do not let the flood sweep over me, or the deep swallow me up, or the Pit close its mouth over me. Answer me, O Lord, for your steadfast love is good; according to your abundant mercy, turn to me. Do not hide your face from your servant, for I am in distress—make haste to answer me.

Psalm 5:2-3

Listen to the sound of my words, O Lord; give heed to my sighing. Listen to the sound of my cry, my King and my God, for to you I pray. O Lord, in the morning you hear my voice; in the morning I plead my case to you, and watch.

Prayer for Trust in Jesus

By St. Ignatius of Loyola

O Christ Jesus,
when all is darkness
and we feel our weakness and helplessness,
give us the sense of your presence,
your love, and your strength.
Help us to have perfect trust
in your protecting love
and strengthening power,
so that nothing may frighten or worry us,
for, living close to you,
we shall see your hand,
your purpose, your will through all things.

Prayer for Understanding

Dear God,
I come to you broken and distraught.
You know my pain, my longing.
All I want is for this ordeal to be over
And to hold a child in my arms.
Help me to stay strong in this struggle,
To refrain from despair and bitterness,
To grow in faith and to wait in hope,
comforted by your care.
We ask this in the name of Jesus. Amen.

Chapter One

Why, God?

*But Abram said, "O Lord God, what will you give me,
for I continue childless?"*

Genesis 15:2

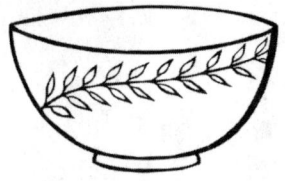

UNTIL INFERTILITY STRUCK, I had the easy, comfortable faith of someone who hasn't suffered much. I was in good health, happily married, well-educated, and working in a job I liked. I'd had a few disappointments along the way, but even those made sense to me as my life unfolded. Having a child seemed like a simple extension of a happy, healthy life.

As we started our journey, I began praying for God to bless us with a healthy child. As the months wore on, my prayers remained quiet and respectful, even as I became alarmed about how long it was taking. In my mind, it was up to God to decide whether we would have children or not. I tried not to question what was happening or do anything that would hurt our chances. In my mind God was like an irritable father home from a bad day at work, and I was his eager-to-please child, careful not to question or upset him.

The spiritual tip-toeing, though, eventually became too much for me to bear. After a while, with so many prayers unanswered, I became angry. Especially on the days when my period came, I would scream and cry, often asking why God was doing this to us. I felt abandoned and alone, as though God were purposefully ignoring my pleas. My anger felt forbidden, but it was a welcome release from the doubts that had begun to creep into my prayers.

As my attitudes changed, I wondered: Who was I to question God's decision? Did I love and trust God only when my prayers were fulfilled? How strong was my belief in God if it fell apart during the first real difficulty I'd had? As I struggled with both infertility and my faith, I couldn't help but think of people who keep their faith alive in the face of chronic pain, crushing poverty, or the loss of a loved one. Here I was, facing the first spiritual crisis of my life, and I felt my own faith turned upside down.

Infertility raises difficult questions, and there are no easy answers. We like to believe that we trust in God's plan even when we don't understand it. But when we encounter something as painful as the struggle to conceive, it is natural to wonder what God is up to. There are no shortcuts through this ordeal. It is hard work to maintain our faith in the midst of suffering. All we can do is be honest and talk with God through prayer, even in our darkest moments.

Anxiety, Anger and Doubt
It took me months to really get angry at God. The anger felt disrespectful and frightening at first, but the longer I ignored my anger, the more it threatened to consume me. I felt passed over by God. Eventually my anger erupted. I screamed at God when my period came. I refused to pray when notions of God came to mind. I had begged God again and again to help us and I was certain God was choosing not to. It felt good to cry and scream, to blame someone for the pain.

Gradually along the way something strange happened. Expressing my anger eventually made me feel closer to God. My image of God had been of some distant spirit far away in the heavens, gauzily granting us our desires in return for obedience. But yelling and screaming made God feel more real, more immediate. It's not easy to rage at someone we don't know, and our strongest feelings—good or bad—are reserved for those we know best. Month by month I began to allow myself to yell at God when I needed to, certain that God could handle a few harsh words. Instead of rote prayers, my time with God began to feel like conversation.

When I was too angry at God, I simply stopped speaking. But after a few days I always found myself returning to our ongoing conversation. In a few grace-filled moments I felt God's presence so keenly that I knew, no matter what happened, God would take care of me. Like my anger, those moments too were fleeting. Soon I was confused and uncertain again, but ultimately those fleeting moments of grace sustained me through my darkest times.

Anger is scary; but for a person of faith undergoing an ordeal like infertility, doubt can be even more frightening.

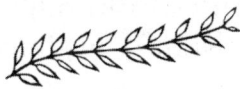

As month after month of prayers go unanswered, we can begin to wonder if God is even there. Anger is scary, but for a person of faith undergoing an ordeal like infertility, doubt can be even more frightening. We begin to question whether our belief in God has been an illusion. We look for signs, reconsider our convictions, and wonder what it all means.

We can't force these moments of doubt out of our minds or shoo them away. They are a normal part of our faith. What we can do is sit in silence and wait for God to respond to us. When we simply can't muster up another prayer, time spent in quiet meditation is a chance for us to reconnect with God. It helps, too, in moments of doubt, to spend time actively seeking examples of God's work in the world. The awe that a sunset inspires, or the comfort of a colleague's kind words, are reminders that a wonderful God has created the world in which we live. If we are open to them, these moments may be enough to sustain us in an otherwise dark time.

How to Pray

We want a child more than anything in the world. Yet we also want—or at least know that we should want—for God's will to be done. What if it's not God's will for us to have a child? What then should we pray for?

This is a difficult issue. After all, Jesus tells the crowd in the Sermon on the Mount: "Ask and it will be given to you; search, and you will find; knock, and the door will be opened for you" (Matthew 7:7). And it's not as though we're asking for a million dollars or a new car. We are asking to obey God's command to be fruitful and multiply. We are asking to work with God in the creation of new life.

In addition, it is difficult for us to pray for something if our heart isn't really in it. Hundreds of times I prayed for God's will to be done—but inside of me a small voice whispered, "And let it be your will that we have a child!"

I believe the answer is simply to keep praying. If our prayer is sincere, God will lead us to an answer. Slowly we may find ourselves asking for things that are in God's plan for us, or we may continue to struggle against God's nudgings. Even just considering the gap between what we want and what God wants for us can help lead us to resolution. And if we pray too long for our own desires, rather than God's, we must know that God understands. God is patient and willing to wait while we figure out how best to pray.

A spiritual challenge such as infertility can open up a world of new prayers, practices and rituals. As I searched for answers to my crisis, I turned to spiritual practices that, as a post-Vatican II Catholic, I had never used before. I began saying the Rosary and found comfort in its rhythms, especially the meditations that encompassed the joyful, sorrowful, glorious and luminous events in Jesus' life. I tried the Lourdes water my aunt sent me. I researched the patron saints of the infertile and made novenas to them.

These rituals can enrich our prayer lives and deepen our faith. But we must be careful. Infertility can leave us vulnerable to practices that are at odds with our faith. We hear of something that worked for the friend of a friend and we seize upon it, even though we know or suspect that it runs counter to what we truly believe.

Once, during a tough time, I stumbled across a novena to St. Clare online that was "guaranteed to work." The petitioner had to recite it every day for nine days, then publish it somewhere, and his or her prayer would be fulfilled. In a moment (okay, nine days) of weakness, I recited it. I even lit the candle that the novena required. And then I waited.

When my period came as usual, I felt a little sheepish. But I was reminded that faith is not magic. A set of words repeated any number of times cannot guarantee a result, no matter how greatly we desire that result. There is nothing wrong with a novena, or a prayer to a patron saint. But these rituals alone are not faith. They are a means to an end, and that end should always be a closer relationship to God.

Turning to Church

For me, one of the hardest times in our struggle with infertility was attending baptisms at our church. The parents in their ties and dresses, the godparents and grandparents beaming, the babies.... I'd remember the baby's mother wasn't even pregnant when we started trying to conceive, and now here she was, a year later, with an infant in her arms, and all I had were mounting medical bills and an unbearable sadness in my heart.

Beyond baptisms, there were First Communions, and children's Masses, and cry rooms, and pregnant women: all reminders of the one thing we wanted most and couldn't seem to grasp. After a while I found myself wanting to skip church because it hurt so much to be there. I know others who ended up leaving their churches altogether, precisely because they felt abandoned during their struggle with infertility. I knew the statistics on infertility—the Centers for Disease Control and

Prevention states that one in six couples of childbearing age are unable to conceive—so I knew by looking around our church that others must be struggling as we were. But their pain, like ours, was silent.

In any other spiritual crisis—the death of a loved one, perhaps, or a cancer diagnosis—most Christians would call their pastors and the people they worship with in search of comfort. But infertility is different. Often churches, instead of providing solace to the infertile, make the condition even more painful for sufferers by reaching out primarily to families with children. And although churches are increasingly adept at confronting a host of modern problems, they don't seem to know quite what to do with those of us struggling with infertility.

Some people also fear hearing that we are somehow to blame for our infertility. We're afraid our infertility is God's will, or a curse we've somehow brought on our-selves. We can find ourselves at odds with the teachings of

Sometimes with just a little effort, we can find solace in our churches.

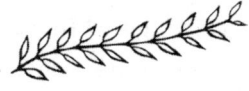

the church we attend. Many Christian denominations teach that at least some infertility treatment is wrong (there is more on this in Chapter 6, "Making Decisions"). When our only option for conceiving is at odds with what our church teaches, many people feel torn and alienated.

When going to church is a source of anxiety and sorrow, many people prefer to stay home and worship

God privately. I don't think anyone would deny us that right, if we feel that's what is best for us. But sometimes with just a little effort, we can find solace in our churches. Many congregations or dioceses have started support groups for the infertile. It's a good idea to check with your local chapter of RESOLVE to see if they know of any (a quick look on an Internet search engine will probably turn up some near you). It often helps to ask people to pray for you, perhaps with a brief explanation that you've been trying to start a family and have run into some trouble. It might be worthwhile to try another church, maybe one that serves more singles and older people. It's often easier to give up and stay home, but sometimes by doing that we deny ourselves the solace we seek.

I clearly remember how difficult it was to sit through Mother's Day services at our church when we were trying to conceive. Many infertile couples find Mother's Day and Father's Day celebrations too painful to attend, with all the attention and praise parents receive publicly on these special days. It's not that these parents don't deserve it; it's just that the red roses and applause that accompany many of these services feel like cruel reminders that we are not yet part of the club of parents, no matter how desperately we want to be. I was all set to skip church one year on Mother's Day when I decided instead to call our pastor and ask him to acknowledge the infertile that Sunday.

I was nervous when I called our pastor. I blurted out a request that the petitions include some mention of infertility. He expressed his sympathy for our plight with a sincerity that set me at ease, and he promised he would do something. That Sunday I paid close attention as he asked our congregation to pray for all the mothers present and far away, living and dead, "as well as those women who long for motherhood." I felt a sense of relief, and triumph, and no small comfort from those words.

Help from Scripture

In our time of need, many of us turn to the Bible and to the women there who struggle with infertility: Sarah, who laughs bitterly when she is told that she will bear a child in her old age; Rachel, who laments that she would rather die than continue living as a barren woman; Elizabeth, whose joyful pregnancy coincides with Mary's; and especially Hannah, mother of Samuel.

Hannah's story was especially meaningful to me as our months of infertility gave way to years. Hannah has a husband who loves her, but it is not enough:

> She wept bitterly. "O Lord of hosts, if only you will look on the misery of your servant, and remember me, and not forget your servant, but will give to your servant a male child, then I will set him before you as a nazirite until the day of his death" (1 Samuel: 1: 10-11).

The priest Eli sees her and mistakes her grief for drunkenness. She explains herself, and he joins in her prayer for a child. Not long after, Hannah and her husband conceive Samuel. She fulfills her promise to dedicate him to God:

> "For this child I prayed; and the Lord has granted me the petition that I made to him. Therefore I have lent him to the Lord, as long as he lives, he is given to the Lord" (1 Samuel: 1:27-28).

I thought of how scared Mary must have been as the angel announced her pregnancy.

I saw my own sadness in Hannah's desperate grief, and I too promised that I would raise any child God granted me to love and serve God.

I also began to view Mary in a different light as I recited my many rosaries. For some time it had been difficult for me to be around pregnant women. Their cheerfully-big bellies aroused an ugly jealousy in me. But as I repeated the Hail Mary again and again, I thought of how scared Mary must have been as the angel announced her pregnancy and how difficult it must have been to tell others about it. I thought of the pregnant women I avoided on the street. How did I know they were happy about their pregnancies? Maybe they were worried about the baby's health, or scared the baby's father would leave. With Mary's help, I began to realize how futile my envy was.

Lessons Learned

I like to think that I took my faith seriously even before infertility. I was always careful to thank God for my many blessings. Looking back now, though, I see that my faith in God reflected too closely the comfortable world in which so many of us live. Although my head told me otherwise, before infertility I believed at some level that I could attain anything I wanted if I worked hard enough. Then that belief came up against the limits of biology. No amount of effort—no homework, no research, no good intentions—could change the fact that my husband and I could not conceive.

It was an important lesson, but a painful one. To this day I struggle with the idea that God is ultimately in control, that there is little I can do to influence what God has already planned for my life. But I know in my soul now that it's true. This knowledge has shaped the way I respond to news of death, illness, and other suffering.

Just as we want to control our own fate, it is human nature to do everything we can to avoid suffering. Even Jesus, facing the painful death he has agreed to accept, asks for reprieve: "If it is possible, let this cup pass from me" (Matthew 26:39). Who among us doesn't do the same as we wonder why we've been singled out for the ordeal of infertility? We promise to attend church faithfully, to raise our child to be a saint, if only God will grant us this one wish.

But Jesus continues: "Yet not what I want, but what you want." Jesus knows, as so many of us discover during a battle with infertility, that we can't avoid suffering.

What we can do is cry as many tears as we need to, allow ourselves to feel the anger and doubt (both of which are natural emotions) and reach out to God and to those around us for comfort.

PRAYER AND REFLECTION

Psalm 13

How long, Lord? Will you forget me forever? How long will you hide your face from me?

How long must I bear pain in my soul, and have sorrow in my heart all day long? How long shall my enemy be exalted over me?

Consider and answer me, O Lord, my God! Give light to my eyes, or I will sleep the sleep of death,

And my enemy will say, "I have prevailed," my foes will rejoice because I am shaken.

I trust in your steadfast love. My heart shall rejoice in your salvation. I will sing to the Lord, because he has dealt bountifully with me.

Infertility Prayer

Good St. Gerard, powerful intercessor before the throne of God, wonder-worker of our day, we call upon you and seek your aid. You know that this marriage has not as yet been blessed with a child and how much [husband's name] and [wife's name] desire this gift. Please present these fervent pleas to the Creator of life from whom all parenthood proceeds and beseech Him to bless this couple with a child whom they may raise as His child and heir of heaven. Amen.

Prayer of Longing

Hear me, O Lord.
Sometimes you feel so far away.
I pray and pray, and I wonder if you hear me.
I know there are no guarantees
that you will grant me what I ask.
I want a child so badly,
But I want too to do your will.
I will try my hardest to trust you,
even when it's hard to do.
All I ask is that you let me feel your presence
And comfort me in these dark days.
I ask this through Jesus Christ, our Lord.
Amen.

In Time of Need

O Lord, this is all my desire—to walk along the path of life that thou hast appointed me, even as Jesus my Lord would walk along it, in steadfastness of faith, in meekness of spirit, in lowliness of heart, in gentleness of love. And because outward events have so much power in scattering my thoughts and disturbing the inward peace in which alone the voice of thy spirit is heard, do thou, gracious Lord, calm and settle my soul by that subduing power which alone can bring all thoughts and desires of the heart into captivity to thyself. All I have is thine; do thou with all as seems best to thy divine will; for I know not what is best. Let not the cares or duties of this life press on me too heavily; but lighten my burden, that I may follow thy way in quietness, filled with thankfulness for thy mercy, and rendering acceptable service unto thee.

Maria Hare (1798-1870)

*We are not necessarily doubting
that God will do the best for us;
we are wondering how painful
the best will turn out to be.*

C. S. Lewis

Chapter Two

Men, Women and Marriage

And be kind to one another,
tender-hearted, forgiving one another.

Ephesians 4:32

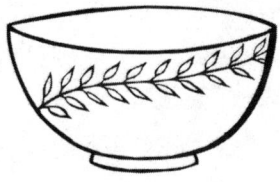

WITHIN THE BIBLICAL STORY OF HANNAH'S quest to conceive, there is a portion that always makes me laugh. Hannah and Elkanah, who go on to become Samuel's parents, have been trying to expand their family for a while. To complicate matters, Elkanah has another wife who's given birth to several children and likes to goad Hannah about it. Hannah is understandably depressed, even despondent. Her husband loves her, even more than he loves his other wife, and tries to cheer her up: "Her husband Elkanah said to her: 'Hannah, why do you weep? Why do you not eat? Why is your heart sad? Am I not more to you than ten sons?'" (1 Samuel 1:8). Hannah runs weeping to the temple to pray once again for a child.

It is a heartbreaking scene, but I always like to imagine Hannah on the phone to her friends afterward: "He doesn't understand why I'm so upset! Doesn't he realize how badly I want this baby? I feel like I'm going through this all by myself!" And Elkanah, talking to his buddy at the gym, no doubt complains, "No matter what I do, it's the wrong thing. I try to cheer her up, tell her how much I love her, and she bites my head off."

We like to think of ourselves, at the dawn of the twenty-first century, as far more enlightened and evolved than people of ancient times. But when it comes to communicating with one another in the midst of infertility, things haven't changed for many couples since the time of Hannah and Elkanah (except for that obnoxious other wife). When we begin our quest for a child, we are united in marriage and in our desire to have children. We try out baby names, throw around hypothetical child-rearing scenarios ("What if our child had a tantrum in the grocery store?"), and generally revel in the joyous journey we are about to make.

But then, gradually or all at once, infertility creeps into our marriage, bringing with it questions, doubts and fears. It silences our light-hearted banter and chips away at our unity. It leaves us at odds with the one person who is best equipped to understand the ordeal we are experiencing. Infertility is a minefield for the happiest of couples, and sometimes the death knell for a shaky relationship. So many enormous decisions to consider, so many potential fights in the making. Is it time to see a specialist, or should we give it a few more months? Are we willing to move onto high-tech treatments? When is it time to end treatment? What about adoption? Should we live without children? It doesn't help that infertility often strikes in the first few years of marriage, when we're still getting to know one another and developing ways to cope with problems. When we promised, on our wedding days, to love one another in sickness, few of us had this particular affliction in mind.

Society promotes stereotypes about how men and women handle crises differently. Women like to talk about their feelings, while men prefer to direct their energy into action. But many times those stereotypes are accurate, and in a crisis like infertility they often become magnified. Even a man who considers himself quite emotionally sensitive may find the easiest way to cope with infertility is by distracting himself with work or hobbies. Many women, meanwhile, seem to deal with their pain by thinking and talking about infertility almost nonstop.

Some of the problems that crop up as a result of infertility in a marriage come from these differences in the way men and women experience the condition, and the trouble we have in communicating those differences. When we can't understand what our partner is feeling, or can't fully explain to our partner what we are feeling, it leads to an even greater sense of isolation. The one person we should be able to lean on becomes instead another source of frustration. Our relationship becomes one more thing to worry about.

Tension enters our marriage in many ways. A man may balk at giving a semen sample at a doctor's request, angering his wife who has endured countless shots, tests and surgery. A woman may be ready to move on to in-vitro fertilization while her husband, worried about the cost, wants to hold off for a while. A man may be uneasy about the notion of adopting even after his wife has fallen in love with a child on an international-adoption web site. Trying to understand the crisis through the perspective of our partner, even when we don't agree with it, can help diffuse the conflicts that infertility creates in a marriage.

There's also a strain on our sex lives. Lovemaking, rather than being a spontaneous act, becomes scheduled. Doctors and nurses quiz us about our most intimate moments. We may become self-conscious about our bodies and resentful of the demands that infertility places on us. Those of us whose physical problems contribute to infertility may feel guilty or wonder if their partners regret marrying them, despite all assurances to the contrary.

Infertility tries the strength of marriage. It can drive a wedge between us and our spouse and leave us guarded around the one person we should be able to trust with our enormous sadness. But through open communication and good will toward one another, infertility can make our marriage stronger and give us the confidence that, no matter what the crisis, we can weather it as a team. I know my marriage was strengthened as a result of our struggle with infertility. Having survived that, I feel like we can face anything together.

Understanding Men and Infertility

Go to any infertility support group and look around. Chances are the crowd will be almost entirely female, with a few sheepish husbands dragged along for support. Visit a website devoted to coping with infertility and it's the same thing: Even the message boards dedicated to men's issues are full of women seeking advice about their husbands. In the offices of reproductive specialists, men often look as though they'd rather be anywhere else, while their wives sit and cry or peruse the thousands of pages of information they've downloaded from the Internet.

Whatever the root of a couple's infertility problem, it must be solved together. But that doesn't mean men and women take equal roles in addressing the problem. For many reasons, women often take the lead in pursuing treatment and researching options. The reasons have to do with the roles that tradition, society and biology assign us, as well as differences in communication styles between men and women. There are exceptions, but these generalizations are common enough to be recognized in the majority of relationships tested by infertility. Understanding them can help us work together, rather than at odds with one another, to reach a resolution.

Most men are, at heart, problem-solvers. Present them with a difficult situation and they want to fix it. Is the door squeaking? Oil it. Feeling underpaid? Ask for a raise. Having trouble conceiving? Just tell them what to do and they'll do it. Women need to remember that most husbands would do anything to give their wives the baby they both desire so much. As one man who was in treatment for infertility said, "I'd build a house out of splinters if I thought it would

Infertility is one problem that can't be fixed merely through hard work and dedication.

help." But this is one problem that can't be fixed merely through hard work and dedication. Infertility is mysterious and frequently hard to fix. It drags on and on, often with a series of specialists who are unable to tell us definitively whether our efforts will work. For someone who wants to do whatever it takes to fix a problem, this uncertainty is beyond frustrating.

And while women love to talk things through, considering every angle, every possible scenario or emotion, many men see this as a waste of time. Hours on the phone with friends don't change the fact that the in-vitro cycle didn't work. A session with a therapist won't bring back a baby who was stillborn. Many men don't see the point in naming a baby who was miscarried at six weeks. They see no benefit to spending hours on the Internet chatting about a potential new cure. They want to move on, take action, and reach a conclusion, whatever that conclusion might be.

In addition, men are often more concerned with the financial cost of treatment. A fertility specialist once told me, "The wives always want to know what the chances for success are, and the husbands always want to know how much it's going to cost." Such concerns may seem crass or insignificant to someone who's determined to have a baby at any cost. But men are raised to worry more about providing and paying the bills, and the prospect of spending tens of thousands of dollars with no guarantee of success understandably makes many of them cringe.

Also, locker-room talk aside, most men aren't brought up to discuss intimate details or even the basics of reproduction with one another. Many women who have an infertility problem are already vaguely aware of it. Perhaps they have always had an irregular menstrual cycle or painful periods, or perhaps they are just at an age when conception becomes more difficult. They tend to feel more comfortable talking about these issues with their friends, which gives them an outlet to cope with the sadness infertility brings.

In contrast, a fertility problem can be a huge blow to a man's ego and a threat to his masculinity. Our society equates potency with virility, and a high sperm count is often seen as something enviable. I cringe when I remember that, before our struggle with infertility, a friend told me that she and her husband had conceived on their first attempt. "Your husband must be so proud!" I replied, in reference to his obvious fertility. Men who venture to tell their friends about their fertility problems sometimes get jokes in response, rather than empathy, which make it harder for them to find support in this difficult time. It's no wonder that men with fertility problems are so often devastated by the discovery.

In addition, the one contribution men make to infertility testing and treatment is often a humiliating one. Providing a semen sample—walking into an office with a small cup and handing it to a (frequently female) technician—is at its core degrading and difficult for most men. Doing it again and again, over the course of a long treatment, doesn't make it any easier. Many women counter that they're the ones who must endure shots, ultrasounds, surgeries, and blood tests, but that does nothing to lessen the difficulty many men have performing their duties. In addition, infertility treatment often requires that couples have intercourse at scheduled times. Many men resent the notion that they must have sex simply because their wives happen to be ovulating that day, and it adds to the pressure infertility places on them. And all the doctors' appointments, with their ultrasounds and stirrups, cause men to associate sex with medical procedures, rather than with love and passion.

Infertility places a great deal of pressure on men to be supportive, provide for their wives, and deal with their own grief, all at the same time. They listen to their wives cry, reassure them that everything will be OK, try to help out around the house—and then are baffled when their wives say they feel like they're going through infertility alone. Men often feel useless; one man I know likened his role to that of a field-goal kicker in a football game, relegated to the sidelines most of the time and then called upon to perform under intense pressure. It's a difficult role they are asked to play. Remembering that can help to diffuse some of the tension that infertility brings to a marriage.

Understanding Women and Infertility

We'll probably never know whether it's nature or nurture that leads girls to play with dolls, but the fact remains that most women grow up fully expecting that we will be mothers someday. Many of us pick out our favorite baby names while we are still in grade school, babysit enthusiastically in high school, and consider careers based on how they would mesh with the demands of child-rearing. And when we meet our future spouses, we consider what sort of fathers they would make, even what our future children would look like.

So when we come up against the limits of our fertility, it is often more than just a physical problem. What's at stake is a lifelong dream, how we see ourselves and what we want our lives to be. We feel betrayed by our bodies and denied the one thing that seems to come so easily to everyone we know. We may respond in different ways, but most women I know become consumed by the quest to have a baby. This determination gives us a sense of control at a time when our bodies, dreams and lives seem out of control.

A woman who is trying to become pregnant is ruled by her body. She must always know what day of her cycle it is and when her period is due. If she's undergoing treatment she must remember when to take her medications, some-times several times a day. She has to call to schedule ap-pointments and juggle work with sometimes daily trips to the doctor's office. When her period is due she may run to the bathroom several times an hour to see whether it has arrived, or obsess about every little twinge she feels in the middle of the night. Add to all this the stress of rapidly-changing hormones and medications that can cause depression, and it's no wonder that some women quit their jobs in order to manage treatments.

A woman who is trying to become pregnant is ruled by her body.

My own personal response was to learn everything I could about reproduction. I spent hours online researching infertility and possible cures, communicating with others through message boards, and considering the advice of specialists from around the country. My research came in handy when I was able to figure out that the first gynecologist we visited was a quack, unable to read my basal body temperature (BBT) chart and convinced that in-vitro fertilization was a waste of time and money (even though most couples who use it are eventually successful). But on our first visit to a respected specialist, when I began rattling off acronyms for little-known hormones and offering advice about specific medications, the doctor told me I had to spend less time online and trust him to make the decisions.

It sounds obvious, but the fact that women are the ones who carry babies in their wombs means that our experience of infertility will always be different than men's. A fetus that died at ten weeks will always be physically abstract to its father, no more than a blob on an ultrasound. But that same baby was a physical part of its mother, who will never forget the stab of fear she felt when she saw the blood that signaled its death. A woman whose doctor tells her she will never become pregnant must mourn the fact that she will never feel a child moving inside her, never experience the pangs of labor, or hear the cry of an infant just born to her. It is a death not only of a dream, but of a real, physical connection that we long for.

Protecting Marriage in the Midst of Infertility
Couples who are confronting infertility can begin to understand one another better by explaining—in a quiet moment over dinner, rather than in the heat of an

argument—exactly how infertility feels to them. Does it feel like it's taking over? Is it a reminder of another difficult time in life? Is it easier to ignore it than think too much about it? There are no right or wrong answers. Simply hearing how it feels to one another is enough at the beginning.

As couples listen to one another, it's important to remember there is no one right way to react to this ordeal. Just because our husbands don't feel the need to talk about it all the time doesn't mean they're not hurting. And a woman who names the fetus she miscarried may be doing what she feels is necessary to move on, even though it seems overwrought to her husband.

Understanding these differences doesn't mean we won't disagree or argue about what we should do in the face of infertility. There are enormous decisions to make as we resolve our infertility, and conflict is a natural part of that process. But many couples find it easier to help one another grieve once we know what our partners are feeling.

It's also helpful for many couples to place limits on the amount of time we spend talking about infertility. If a woman knows that for fifteen minutes every evening she can talk about her fears and questions, she's likely to feel that she's being heard. And her husband, knowing the discussion won't go on forever, is more likely to participate and listen actively.

Remember too, that both spouses in a marriage tested by infertility are grieving. No matter what the circumstances or reasons, whether we obsess about it all the time or act like nothing's happening, we are both in pain because of the disease. By working harder to comfort our spouse, we often come to spend less time wondering why he or she isn't grieving the way we do.

It also helps many couples to look at infertility the way we'd look at a cancer diagnosis or another medical crisis. Often in the face of illness, couples unite against the common enemy that is disrupting our lives. Although infertility is fraught with emotional baggage that few other diseases carry, it is in the end a disease, and couples who are united against it stand a better chance of overcoming it.

Couples who are united against infertility stand a better chance of overcoming it.

And while married couples need to rely on one another, we also need to find other people to support us during this difficult time. The grief from infertility is at times so overwhelming that no one person can provide all the comfort and support that his or her partner needs. Professional help from a minister or therapist—for both couples and individuals—is an excellent way to help cope with this pain. I found it helpful to seek out couples who also were suffering from infertility, because no one better understood what we were going through than two people who were walking the same road.

Happy marriages need fun and recreation to thrive. We must take time to enjoy one another's company, even in the midst of conflict or grueling treatment. Go away for a weekend, try a new restaurant, or just take a bath together, and promise not to talk about infertility for the duration of your time together. And take time to enjoy one another's bodies and the gift of lovemaking—not merely as a means to the much-desired end of conception, but as a wonderful gift from God and a great source of pleasure.

Finally, remember that as we try so hard to conceive, we already have a family that deserves nurturing and care. When we were first married, my husband Erik often referred to "our family" when talking about the two of us. "We need to do what's best for our family," he'd say when trying to decide how to spend a bonus or when to plan a vacation. At first I was puzzled and looked around the room to see who else he was talking about. Gradually, though, and especially after we began our struggle with infertility, I began to see the wisdom of his point of view. We already were a family, whether we had children or not. And as we tried to add children to the mix, we had to take special care not to jeopardize the sacred relationship at the heart of our family.

PRAYER AND REFLECTION

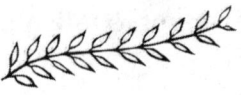

1 Corinthians 13:4-7
Love is patient; love is kind; love is not envious or boastful or arrogant or rude. It does not insist on its own way; it is not irritable or resentful; it does not rejoice in wrongdoing, but rejoices in the truth. It bears all things, believes all things, hopes all things, endures all things.

Ecclesiastes 4:9-11
Two are better than one because they have a good reward for their toil. For if they fall, one will lift up the other; but woe to one is alone and falls and does not have another to help. Again, if two lie together, they keep warm; but how can one keep warm alone?

Spouses' Prayer for One Another

Lord Jesus,
grant that I and my spouse may have a true
and understanding love for one another.
Grant that we may both
be filled with faith and trust.
Give us the grace to live
with one another in peace and harmony.
May we always bear with one another's weaknesses
and grow from one another's strengths.
Help us to forgive one another's failings
and grant us patience, kindness, cheerfulness
and the spirit of placing the well-being
of one another ahead of self.

May the love that brought us together
grow and mature with each passing year.
Bring us both ever closer to You
through our love for one another.
Let our love grow to perfection.

Prayer of an Infertile Couple

Dear God,
United in love, we want so much to conceive a child,
A child who would reflect the love we have for one
another,
A child whom we would raise to love and worship You.
Yet so far, our efforts are in vain,
And each disappointing month brings us more sadness.
We ask You, God, if it is Your will,
To grant us the child we both want so much.
And we ask you too to help us care for one another
As we endure this trial;
To be kind to one another,
To take time for one another,
To remember the love that unites us with You.
We ask this in Jesus' name.
Amen.

Prayer for Marriage

Most gracious God, we give you thanks for your tender love in sending Jesus Christ to come among us, to be born of a human mother, and to make the way of the cross to be the way of life.

We thank you, also, for consecrating the union of man and woman in his Name.

By the power of your Holy Spirit, pour out the abundance of your blessing upon this man and this woman.

Defend them from every enemy.

Lead them into all peace.

Let their love for one another be a seal upon their hearts, a mantle about their shoulders, and a crown upon their foreheads.

Bless them in their work and in their companionship; in their sleeping and in their waking; in their joys and in their sorrows; in their life and in their death.

Finally, in your mercy, bring them to that table where your saints feast for ever in your heavenly home; through Jesus Christ our Lord, who with you and the Holy Spirit lives and reigns, one God, for ever and ever. Amen.

Book of Common Prayer (1979)

Chapter Three

The Isolation of Infertility

Be strong and bold; have no fear or dread of them,
because it is the Lord your God who goes with you;
he will not fail you or forsake you.

Deuteronomy 31:6

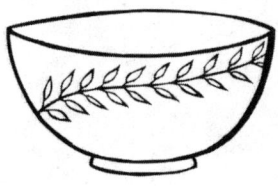

WHEN WE ARE IN THE MIDST OF INFERTILITY, the world is a minefield of pregnant women and cherubic babies. The receptionist at work is due any day now; a friend or neighbor calls to give us the good news that they're expecting; a trip through the mall turns up newborns and strollers around every corner. Every day brings painful reminders that we are unable to conceive, even though it seems to come so easily to the rest of the world.

Even when we manage to avoid pregnant women and newborns, we encounter friends and relatives with their questions and unwanted advice. We cringe as they ask us when we're going to start a family or advise us to just "relax and take a vacation." Even strangers unwittingly remind us of our feelings of failure. Again and again, I remember people asking me how many children I had. I always sighed a bit as I replied "none," hoping the person I was talking to wouldn't follow up with any more intrusive questions.

One of the saddest aspects of infertility is that it isolates us from the people around us at the exact moment when we most need love and support. People we'd turn to in any other crisis can't fully understand the pain we're feeling. Our relationships with friends who have children can become strained simply because it's difficult to be around them. Our family members sometimes alienate us with questions and unwanted advice. We struggle with how private our pain should be and whom we should reach out to.

But we can make this difficult time a little easier, for ourselves and those around us, if we know what bothers us most and decide how best to respond. There is no one right way to do this. Each one of us is different, and a comment that might reduce one person to tears may simply roll off the back of another. By taking the time to figure out who or what pains us the most—whether it's an intrusive neighbor or workplace baby showers— we can take some pressure off ourselves and make this difficult time a little easier. That doesn't mean ending a friendship with a couple that's expecting; it simply means a little time away while we sort out our options.

And while other people can be a source of pain for the infertile, they can also be a source of great comfort and peace if they have been through the same ordeal. Reaching out to others who are now facing infertility, or who have dealt with it in the past, is perhaps the single best way to combat our feelings of isolation. When we meet and talk to others we learn how common the struggle to have children is. We draw strength from the stories of other people and the many happy resolutions they've reached. We realize that we too will someday resolve our own infertility, though we may not know exactly how just yet.

Living in the Fertile World

Is there any event more painful for someone who's infertile than a baby shower? The glowing parents-to-be; the adorable clothes and toys; the grandparents beaming with pride; the excitement on the faces of the guests. In the midst of my infertility, I attended showers with a knot in my stomach. I was happy for my friends and wished them nothing but the best. But it was excruciating to sit through a baby shower with all the women recalling their own pregnancies and all the men making jokes about college funds. It made me feel envious and petty and, worst of all, like a complete failure. I always went because I thought I should, but I spent most of my time fighting back tears.

It's not just baby showers that can be difficult. Friends call from the hospital, inviting us to come see their new-borns. Our neighbors invite us to their toddler's birthday party. A group of friends who all have children ask us to attend a holiday party that will be packed with babies. We wonder: Should we go and risk upsetting ourselves, or avoid the happy families and risk offending our friends?

Should we go and risk upsetting ourselves, or avoid the happy families and risk offending our friends?

After much thought and prayer, I've concluded that for those of us coping with infertility, taking care of our own needs is paramount. We must know the situations that are upsetting and painful—and avoid them. We want to seem happy for our loved ones, and under normal circumstances we would be. But for now, their excitement only underscores our own disappointment. If we don't feel up to visiting a newborn in the hospital, or attending a co-worker's shower, it's acceptable to simply not go. We can call and say we can't make it—no explanation necessary—then go out and do something nice for ourselves.

That doesn't mean ignoring a loved one's happy occasion. Sending a card and a gift is often easier and less risky than fighting back tears at a large gathering. If our friends truly love us, they know that their happiness is a reminder of our pain, and they are willing to forego our company if it means protecting our feelings. Sometimes crises like infertility reveal a person's true character, and a friend who is upset at us for not attending a shower or a party may not in the end be a friend at all.

Can we be friends with people who are expecting or have small children? Of course it's possible, but in this difficult time we need to take care of ourselves first. Sometimes our relationships are so solid that we can share our pain with our friends and feel uplifted by them, even when they are celebrating something we long for so deeply. Other times we need a break from our friendships, perhaps until our infertility is resolved. And still other relationships are damaged irreparably as a result of infertility. There is no right or wrong answer when it comes to these questions. We can only listen to our hearts and pray for the guidance to honor our friends as we protect ourselves.

The Problem of Envy

It's worth thinking a bit more about how we may envy fertile people while we are struggling with infertility.

There is no feeling quite so awful as envy—especially when the object of our envy is an innocent infant or a beaming, expectant parent. It makes us feel petty and mean, guilty and ashamed. It's embarrassing to acknowledge (even to ourselves) and difficult to talk about with others. If we consider ourselves religious or spiritual people, those pangs of pregnancy or baby envy probably make us feel guilty or shameful. The Bible, and Christian tradition, warn of the dangers of jealousy and condemn it forcefully: "A tranquil mind gives life to the flesh, but passion makes the bones rot" (Proverbs 14:30). Envy is the only emotion that shows up in both the Ten Commandments and the Seven Deadly Sins; isn't that proof that we shouldn't be feeling it?

If our struggles with infertility have made us envious of others, it's best first off to cut ourselves some slack. The urge to have a child is powerful, both biologically and psychologically, and finding out that it might not be possible creates an enormous crisis for most people. Envy is a natural part of this crisis. The happiness of others is a constant reminder of what we want and don't yet have.

Envy may be a natural and normal reaction to infertility, but that's not to say it's healthy or good for us. Infertility can quickly become all-consuming. When we long for a baby more than anything in the world, it's easy to convince ourselves that our lives are worthless without a baby, that if we just had one then everything would be okay. When we do this, we risk overlooking all the gifts that God has given us.

In Genesis, Rachel laments that she will die if she does not have children. Although it sounds melodramatic, many of us recognize the pain and desperation in Rachel's cry. So it might upset us to read the next line: "Jacob became very angry with Rachel and said, 'Am I in the place of God, who has withheld from you the fruit of the womb?'" (Genesis 30:2).

Sure, Jacob sounds like an insensitive and uncaring oaf. But consider for a moment all the advantages Rachel has. Both she and her sister Leah are married to Jacob, but Rachel is considered the more beautiful of the two. Jacob loves her more. In fact, Jacob was tricked into marrying Leah, thinking she was Rachel, and he waited around another seven years in order to marry Rachel.

Yet Rachel is not thankful for Jacob's love, nor for her great beauty. Instead she sees life as a competition between herself and her sister. God consoles Leah for being unloved by giving her four sons. Rachel remains childless, and for this reason she wants to die. She thinks of herself only in terms of childbearing ability, not as an intellectual or moral being capable of great love. It's easier to understand Jacob's anger (if not his exact choice of words) when we consider her envy more carefully.

And while Rachel envies Leah for being able to bear children, Leah in turn envies Rachel because Jacob loves Rachel more. One of Leah's sons finds some mandrakes, which were believed to promote fertility, and Rachel asks for them. Leah responds, "Is it a small matter that you have taken away my husband? Would you take away my son's mandrakes also?" Leah is clearly in pain, and her children are insufficient consolation for the inadequacy she feels around her sister.

We are all unique beings, created in the image of God, with gifts we are supposed to use for God's glory. Some people have careers we love, or a close and loving family; others have artistic talents or a knack for making people feel at ease. Whatever our talents, God gave them to us with the hope that we would use them to their fullest. If we put our lives on hold until we have a child, we are neglecting our precious gifts. Sometimes it helps to make a list of things healthy and fruitful in our lives, and keep it close as a reminder during our weak moments.

If we put our lives on hold until we have a child, we are neglecting our precious gifts.

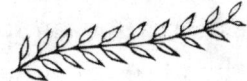

There are even treasures to find in the midst of our pain. Often a marriage is strengthened by the ordeal of infertility. (If so, thank God for that.) Or maybe our friends have been even more supportive than usual. We can learn patience and empathy as we wait for our family to grow.

This isn't meant to minimize the pain of infertility. There are few things in life that hurt more than wanting a baby and not being able to have one. If we are feeling low and sorry for ourselves, it can be soothing to give in to the pangs of envy for a moment. But remember that allowing envy to flourish goes against God's wishes for us. Like hate or anger, it divides us rather than unites us, and it makes us competitors when we should be supporters of one another.

There is also a futility to envy, because we can never know what the lives of the people we envy are really like. Consider someone who stares at or avoids contact with pregnant women or infants. This is natural and normal, but it is also a waste of time and energy. That pregnant woman on the bus may be fearful that her boyfriend will leave once the baby is born. Maybe that couple in the mall, cooing over their newborn, adopted her after years of unsuccessful fertility treatments. Or maybe the strangers are having easy pregnancies that were carefully planned—the point is, we don't know anything about their lives, so what good is it to envy them?

When I was in treatment for infertility, I began saying the Rosary, and naturally began thinking more and more about Mary. I began to wonder if I would have envied Mary had I seen her on the street during her pregnancy. And that led me to contemplate how scared she must have been as the angel proclaimed her pregnancy, and how difficult it must have been to tell others—starting with her fiancé, Joseph—about it.

I thought of the pregnant women I saw (and avoided) on the street. Their reproductive success had nothing to do with my failure. It wasn't as though I'd get pregnant if only somehow they weren't. With Mary's help, I began to realize how futile my envy was.

Friends and Family

It's not just expectant couples we tend to avoid when we're dealing with infertility. Co-workers, cousins, even people at the gym seem to have an inexhaustible supply of nosy questions and awkward comments.

When are you two going to fill up that house? You're not getting any younger, you know."

"Your husband is so good with babies. When are you going to have some of your own?"

"You guys want kids? Honestly, you can take mine. They're driving me crazy!"

"You're having trouble getting pregnant? You guys need any help?"

It's easy to shake our heads and even laugh at these comments when we're rehashing them at home with our spouse. But what do we say when someone blurts one out at coffee hour after church? Some people find it helpful to formulate a response ahead of time to be ready for such questions and comments, especially the really obnoxious ones. But most of us simply smile politely and stifle the impulse to answer in the meanest way we know how.

The awkwardness we feel over such questions is compounded by the fact that most infertile people don't feel comfortable talking about their condition with others. For many of us, it's hard to let our friends and families see us in a vulnerable state. It's not just infertility; people are often ashamed to tell friends we've lost our job or been rejected from a school we wanted to attend. We want people to be proud of us. Allowing friends or relatives see us when we're down is not always easy to do.

Letting people know that we're struggling to conceive seems especially hard because it's so private and personal. It's such a roller-coaster ride of emotions. When my husband and I first ran into trouble conceiving, I didn't want to tell anyone because I believed we'd be able to resolve it quickly. Then months stretched into years of hope followed by disappointment. I wanted to share our difficulties with those close to us, but I was embarrassed. It wasn't until after I became pregnant that I felt comfortable telling people about the ordeal we'd been through.

Letting people know the source of our pain can be cathartic for us and educational for them.

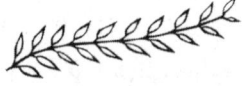

There are times that I regret staying silent so long about our troubles. Sometimes acknowledging our pain to loved ones, however briefly, eases some of the strain that both they and we feel. Infertility remains such a secret shame, even in our talk-show culture, that letting people know the source of our pain can be cathartic for us and educational for them.

I missed out on the chance to educate our friends and relatives about infertility and to help them avoid making insensitive comments to others. I also probably missed making connections with people who were enduring the same struggle, or who had already been through infertility and could have provided some comfort.

Those close to us want us to be happy, and most would be deeply sympathetic and compassionate about our struggle with infertility. By choosing not to talk about it, we are reinforcing the idea that infertility is shameful and embarrassing. As someone who chose not to share much about our difficulty conceiving, I now wish I'd been more open with people. It's an intensely personal decision, though, and one that we need to make again and again until our infertility is resolved.

Working and Infertility
Infertility and its treatment often feel like a part-time job. There are doctors' appointments, trips to the pharmacy, shots and medication that need to be timed just right, phone calls with insurance companies, and other time-consuming tasks. For many people, the work of infertility can interfere with performance at their other, full-time job.

Some people find it easier to stop work altogether during intensive infertility treatment, while others need the distraction of a job to keep them from dwelling on the stress.

I remember when I was going through treatment, I worked in an open space and shared a desk with another person. I didn't want anyone to hear my phone calls to my doctor, so I went downstairs—sometimes several times a day—to use the pay phone in the lobby. How strange it must have looked to anyone who knew me.

Another time I had an opportunity for an overseas business trip, something I really wanted to do. But it was scheduled right at the most fertile time of my cycle, and I didn't want to waste another month's opportunity. My lack of enthusiasm angered my boss, but I didn't feel comfortable telling her why I didn't want to go.

There's no easy solution to dealing with the stress that infertility brings, and no clear formula for deciding how much to tell co-workers and how much to withhold. Many women are reluctant to tell their bosses about their situation because a potential pregnancy could raise the question of how long the employee will stay at the company. On the other hand, if an in-vitro fertilization (IVF) cycle means arriving late every other morning for weeks at a time, it might be best to give a supervisor a heads-up.

And while pregnant friends and relatives are easy to avoid, there's nothing anyone can do to avoid a pregnant co-worker or a visit from an officemate on maternity leave. It's often easiest to find an ally in the office to lean on in difficult times—someone to run interference when the guy down the hall brings his new baby in, or provide a shield when the boss is passing around her daughter's ultrasound pictures. We spend so much time in our work environment, and often form such close relationships there. Many of us can find comfort as well, if we just know where to look for it.

Reaching Out

While undergoing in-vitro fertilization treatment, my husband and I joined a support group sponsored by the medical clinic we were going to. It was a huge relief to be able to cry, commiserate and even laugh with others who were undergoing the same ordeal. Sharing our story with them helped to ease our burden. Hearing their stories, I no longer felt isolated in our suffering.

These relationships, whether in an organized support group or more informally with friends and acquaintances, are perhaps the best way to deal with the pain of infertility. Acknowledging and talking about our feelings somehow makes them easier to accept. By sharing with someone who's been there, we don't have to worry about appearing petty or pathetic. If someone's had even a short bout with infertility, they understand what we're feeling. It may not make our pain disappear, but it's reassuring to know other people feel it.

Several studies have shown that fertility patients who participate in support groups suffer less depression and anxiety and may even have higher pregnancy rates. Group therapy also provides benefits to those seeking treatment for infertility. It's important to note that while infertility often contributes to depression and anxiety, most researchers believe that psychological distress is a result of infertility rather than a cause. Despite the advice to "just relax" that so many of us receive, infertility is usually caused by physical factors rather than by depression or anxiety.

There are many places to find people who understand this particular pain. Nearly everyone knows someone who's faced infertility. Some doctors' offices sponsor support groups for their patients; some churches organize sessions to help members deal with infertility, although some people are reluctant to attend for fear we'll run into someone we know but haven't yet told. Most cities have chapters of the group RESOLVE which sponsors support groups and information sessions for infertility patients.

I always found excellent resources online, in message boards and chat rooms. The anonymity of the Internet makes it a good first choice for finding other people with whom to share the pain of infertility. Typing a few key words into a search engine will bring up many options. However, as comforting as it can be to "meet" people under the guise of Internet anonymity, I found it was important at some point to talk with a real human being. There's a comfort in seeing the pain in another person's face or sharing a laugh that online resources can't provide.

Finally, a pastor or a mental-health professional is a good idea if sadness seems persistent or overwhelming. Up to half of all fertility patients suffer from serious depression stemming from the fact that one of their life's dreams is as of yet unfulfilled, despite all their work to make it come true. Meeting with a professional can help us understand these feelings of loss and give us strength in this time of great need.

PRAYER AND REFLECTION

Isaiah 41:10-13
Do not fear, for I am with you, do not be afraid, for I am your God; I will strengthen you, I will help you, I will uphold you with my victorious right hand. Yes, all who are incensed against you shall be ashamed and disgraced; those who strive against you shall be as nothing and shall perish. You shall seek those who contend with you, but you shall not find them; those who war against you shall be as nothing at all. For I, the Lord your God, hold your right hand; it is I who say to you, "Do not fear, I will help you."

Romans 12:9-15
Let love be genuine, hate what is evil, hold fast to what is good; love one another with mutual affection, outdo one another in showing honor. Do not lag in zeal, be ardent in spirit, serve the Lord. Rejoice in hope, be patient in suffering, preserve in prayer. Contribute to the needs of the saints; extend hospitality to strangers. Bless those who persecute you; bless and do not curse them. Rejoice with those who rejoice; weep with those who weep.

Prayer of St. Francis

Lord, make me an instrument of your peace.
Where there is hatred, let me sow love,
Where there is injury, pardon
Where there is doubt, faith,
Where there is despair, hope,
Where there is darkness, light,
Where there is sadness, joy.
O Divine Master, grant that I may not so much
seek to be consoled as to console,
not so much to be understood as to understand,
not so much to be loved, as to love;
for it is in giving that we receive,
it is in pardoning that we are pardoned,
it is in dying that we awake to eternal life.

Prayer for Patience

Dear God,
My friends disappoint me.
My family frustrates me.
It's so hard to endure this ordeal
And sometimes the people around me
Make it even harder.

Give me the patience to
Breathe deeply when I want to scream;
To speak up when I want to hide;
To utter a kind word when
A mean-spirited one is on my lips.
Help me too to have the courage
To share my struggle
And allow those around me
To lighten my load.

We ask this through Christ our Lord.
Amen.

Chapter Four

Loving Ourselves as God Loves Us

Do not fear, for I am with you, do not be afraid,
for I am your God; I will strengthen you,
I will help you, I will uphold you
with my victorious right hand.

Isaiah 41:10

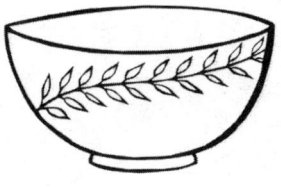

ON THE DARK DAYS when infertility threatens to consume us, it's easy to be hard on ourselves. If only we'd gotten married sooner... If only we'd gone to the doctor earlier... If only I could relax and stop trying so hard to conceive. Sometimes we feel ourselves changing in ways we don't particularly like: withdrawing from life, avoiding other people, sinking into pessimism and gloom as our efforts to conceive drag on.

It probably comes as no surprise that many people experiencing infertility become depressed and anxious. One study found that over half of infertile women considered their infertility to be the single most upsetting experience of their lives; 10 percent fit the definition for major depression; and roughly a third to half reported symptoms of depression. The women surveyed had levels of anxiety and depression equal to women with cancer, HIV or heart disease.

There are many circumstances that make this sense of anxiety and failure even more acute. Some people wonder if we're being punished for a sin or failing that happened long ago. People whose physical problems cause infertility can feel less attractive and may wonder if our spouses regret marrying us. Others, especially women who are over thirty-five, feel old when we see the statistics about how fertility changes over time. Milestones such as birthdays and holidays become painful reminders of the passage of time instead of happy occasions worth celebrating.

Sometimes it helps to remember that people who

can't conceive are grieving as surely as someone who's just lost a loved one is grieving. In many ways, the grief of the infertile is more painful, because our grief starts anew every month when the dream of conception dies yet again. Allowing ourselves to grieve as much as we need to—through rituals, tears, or time off work—will help us gradually accept our loss.

So will remembering that God loves us unconditionally, no matter what we've done, no matter how old we are, no matter the condition of our bodies. We are children of God. We are loved deeply by our Creator. Believing it won't take away all our pain, but it can give us the strength to see ourselves the way God sees us, and to lovingly care for ourselves in this difficult time.

Healing from Past Sin

For some people, the struggle to conceive reminds them of a past hurt, sin or failing. Perhaps it was an abortion, or a child placed for adoption after an unplanned pregnancy, or a long-ago extramarital affair. Or maybe nothing as dramatic as that—just a deeply-held belief that suffering is the result of our own sin. But no matter what we have done, no matter what sorts of skeletons live in our closets, infertility is never a punishment from God. God doesn't work that way; Jesus tells us so when he heals the blind man in the Gospel of John (John 9:1-5).

Jesus' disciples ask if the man is blind because of his own sins or his parents' sins. Jesus answers that neither the man nor his parents are to blame for the man's blindness: The man is blind so that God can work a miracle in his life and thus convince him and others to believe. "Neither he nor his parents sinned;" Jesus says. "It is so that the works of God might be made visible through him" (John 9:3).

So it is with infertility. It is not a punishment for something we've done. It is a chance for God to work in our lives. In one person's life infertility may be a call to start a support group at church. In another it may lead to working for a group that helps women in crisis pregnancies. Maybe it's simply a chance to pause and reflect more deeply on how we can be Jesus to the people we encounter every day. But it is never God's way of punishing us.

> **Infertility is not a punishment for something we've done. It is a chance for God to work in our lives.**

For those who are troubled by past sin in their lives, there are many ways to seek forgiveness. People who are recovering from the effects of abortion, no matter how far in the past, can find groups such as Project Rachel to help them heal. There are also excellent resources on the Internet, and many of them are anonymous, which allows for a safe way to begin healing. More information is available by typing "healing from abortion" or a similar phrase into an Internet search engine.

God forgives us for any sin if we simply ask. And once God has forgiven us, we must forgive ourselves.

Worrying about sins in the past, or believing that infertility is a punishment, can be a diversion from the work that we need to do to heal our bodies and find resolution to this physical ailment.

Healing from Physical Problems

According to the Centers for Disease Control and Prevention, women whose mothers took the medication DES when they were pregnant sometimes have trouble conceiving or carrying an infant to term. Men who have had testicular cancer are often left sterile by the treatment used to save their lives. Diseases such as polycystic ovarian syndrome or endometriosis can also make it difficult for couples to conceive.

The first thing doctors do when a couple comes in for treatment is to try and pinpoint the exact problem or problems preventing conception. According to the American Society for Reproductive Medicine, about one-third of cases can be attributed to the female partner, and another one-third to the male partner. The remaining cases are either a combination of male and female problems or can't be explained.

Finding out the cause is an important first step. But it can also prompt feelings of guilt and shame in those whose bodies are preventing conception. We feel inadequate or unattractive; some even wonder if our spouses are disappointed they married us. Those with chronic illnesses often feel that our bodies are betraying us yet again. We may resent that a serious illness such as cancer continues to haunt us.

A diagnosis of infertility can and should prompt us to take better care of ourselves. Everyone trying to conceive—whether man or woman—should eat a healthy diet, get an adequate amount of sleep, and exercise regularly. Because obesity can contribute to infertility, it also makes sense to try to reach or maintain a healthy weight. Taking care of our bodies not only helps us endure the physical demands of infertility, it also improves our mental health and makes it easier to withstand the unpredictability of the disease.

Beyond this, we are wrong to think less of ourselves simply because of a condition. Patients with cancer or influenza generally don't blame themselves for their sickness, and neither should people who have difficulty conceiving. The reasons for disease are often a mystery, but physical disease is never a punishment from God.

Furthermore, once we've received a diagnosis, it doesn't really matter whose body is responsible for the infertility. We vow on our wedding days to love one another in sickness and in health, and this is the time to live that vow rather than turn on one another. Infertile couples need to battle the disease together by uniting in determination rather than dissolving into blame.

Infertility and Depression
People who are trying to conceive often hear the same well-meaning advice from friends and family members: "Just relax. You're thinking about it too much. My friends went on vacation after years of trying to get pregnant and that's all it took!"

This makes some people wonder if their mental state can make it harder to achieve pregnancy. Can we sabotage our chances of conceiving if we are depressed, anxious, or simply thinking about it too much?

While there's plenty of evidence that infertility causes depression, the research is mixed on whether depression causes or contributes to infertility. Certainly men and women who are depressed or anxious manage to conceive all the time, so it's not as though depression absolutely prevents conception. However, some studies of patients undergoing in-vitro fertilization have found that patients who report a great deal of stress have lower pregnancy rates than patients with lower levels of stress, which indicates emotions might play at least a small role in fertility.

Can we sabotage our chances of conceiving if we are depressed, anxious, or simply thinking about it too much?

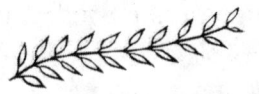

This isn't to suggest that infertile people who are depressed are to blame for their difficulty conceiving. Infertility is a complex affliction, and despite all of our medical advances we still know so little about its causes and cures. But it makes sense for people who are trying to conceive to be in the best mental and emotional shape possible, whether to boost conception rates or simply make it easier to withstand the ups and downs of the fertility rollercoaster.

There's no single best way to improve one's outlook

during infertility. For some people the answer lies in couples' therapy; others prefer seeing a therapist alone. Support groups are a great way to meet other people going through the same ordeal. Exercise, meditation and favorite hobbies are all great ways to relieve tension and stress. I found that the meditative rhythms of the Rosary gave me great comfort while I was undergoing treatment. Whatever the method of coping, it's important to find one that works and use it as often as needed. Infertility is hard enough as it is; whatever we can do to make it easier day-to-day will help us on the road to resolution.

Infertility and Aging
One of the primary reasons for the increase in infertility in recent decades is that people are waiting until later in their lives to have children. There are excellent reasons for this. Women have more educational and career opportunities than ever before, leading them to wait until their schooling is over or their careers are established before they have children. And couples who delay childbearing often make excellent parents. They are more patient and better prepared to make the necessary sacrifices that children inevitably require.

But these couples often face more difficulty conceiving, especially once the female partner reaches her mid-thirties. It is a cruel paradox that when many people finally feel psychologically and economically ready to have children, their physical capacity to conceive is in steep decline.

There's nothing like a trip to a fertility clinic to make

someone—especially a woman—feel old. A woman who is thirty-six or thirty-eight may feel and look even better than she did in her twenties, but in the eyes of a fertility specialist, she is old. She's no doubt already heard all the alarming reports about the drop-off in fertility women experience after age thirty-five, along with the jokes about the biological clocks ticking loudly. No matter what kind of shape she's in or how good she feels, it's going to be hard to walk out of the doctor's office without feeling like damaged goods.

This evidence that we are growing older is a difficult thing to accept in a culture that worships youth and physical vigor. Every day advertisements tell us we can cover our gray, fight our wrinkles, tone our bodies, look ten years younger. We are used to the idea that any sign of aging can be reversed, but no amount of effort can reverse the effects of aging on our reproductive systems.

For many women, infertility is their first evidence that they are growing older. For me, infertility led to a slowly-dawning realization of my own mortality. I always knew on some level that I would die, but now I was faced with physical evidence that my body was growing older and that soon I would be too old to bear children, that I would be middle-aged, that someday this body of mine would cease to work altogether.

I know this sounds depressing, but this knowledge can be liberating as well. We can credit our bout with infertility for helping us to better understand our mortality. Knowing our time here is finite can lead us to re-examine our purpose here on Earth. It can prompt us to ponder more deeply the mystery of creation and God's promise of salvation, and help us to resolve to spend our time here in pursuit of greater meaning. We may resolve to write that book we've always daydreamed about writing, or finally read the Bible from beginning to end, or change careers so that we spend our time in a more fulfilling way. Infertility is a painful way to learn this, but if we are open to its lessons we can find our lives immeasurably enriched because of it.

This passage can also lead us to focus more closely on what it is that makes us worthy of God's infinite love. God doesn't love us because we are young, or in good shape. He doesn't love us because we are intelligent or outgoing or athletic or fertile. God loves us despite our age, our body type, our shyness or clumsiness or infertility. And in loving us unconditionally, God gives us something to strive for: We must try to love others just as God loves us. That means loving our co-worker despite the stupid things he says sometimes. It means loving our parents no matter how much they frustrate us; loving our siblings no matter how distant they sometimes seem; loving the gossipy neighbor and the busybody at church and everyone else we come across. Infertility teaches us that we aren't perfect. God teaches us that no one else is either, but God loves us all, just the same.

Infertility and Time

Whether we are younger or older, infertility changes our relationship with time. For instance, the days in my cycle became more important to me than the days of the month. I didn't always know without looking at the calendar whether it was January 21 or 22, but I always knew, from the moment I awoke in the morning, that it was day 17 of my cycle. Our lives become controlled by the cycle calendar. Lovemaking must be scheduled, and the quest for conception squelches all spontaneity. The cycles take on a depressing similarity as time marches on: beginning with hope, proceeding through anxiety, and usually ending in disappointment.

Milestones take on a different meaning too as we strive to overcome infertility. For the infertile, a birthday becomes yet another reminder that time is passing and we are still without a child in our lives. Thanksgiving and Christmas can be excruciating—all the family get-togethers with nieces and nephews, expectant siblings and in-laws, and the adorable baby Jesus in the manger scene. And Mother's Day—it's no wonder many infertile women just stay home and avoid the red roses and applause that many churches give to mothers in May.

You may notice your prayer life mirroring the cycles of your quest for conception—hopeful at first, then anxious, then despairing. Although frustrating, these cycles can also put us in touch with the rhythms of life—stillness and action, listening and decision. As they become familiar, we can anticipate our emotions and even take comfort in their familiarity. We can also be attuned to changes in our reactions—perhaps when we feel ready to pursue another path, opening our hearts to a different treatment or adoption or something else we weren't ready to consider before.

Contemplative prayer and keeping a journal are excellent ways to experience these rhythms. I find it helpful to practice the two together, in order. In contemplative prayer we meditate and quietly open ourselves to God. We keep quiet and let God do the talking. In silence we can hear what God wants for us, as well as what we want for ourselves. It's best to carve out some time every day for contemplation and meditation. God doesn't always talk to us when we want God to, but by making silent prayer a part of our daily lives, we prepare ourselves to hear God's message when it comes.

Keeping a journal is also a good way to figure out what God wants us to do and what we're prepared to take on. As long as our thoughts and prayers are in our heads, we aren't beholden to them; seeing them on a piece of paper helps us to confront them. In order to hear what God wants for us, and to know what we want for ourselves, it's important to spend as much time listening as writing.

PRAYER AND REFLECTION

John 9:1-3

As (Jesus) walked along, he saw a man blind from birth. His disciples asked him, "Rabbi, who sinned, this man or his parents, that he was born blind?" Jesus answered, "Neither this man nor his parents sinned; he was born blind so that God's works might be revealed in him."

Psalm 25:16-21

Turn to me and be gracious to me, for I am lonely and afflicted. Relieve the troubles of my heart, and bring me out of my distress. Consider my affliction and my trouble, and forgive my sins. Consider how many are my foes, and with what violent hatred they hate me. O guard my life and deliver me; do not let me be put to shame, for I take refuge in you. May integrity and uprightness preserve me, for I wait for you.

God, Remind Me of Your Love

Dear God,
On those days when I feel like a failure,
Old or unhealthy,
A disappointment most of all to myself,
Remind me of your love.
Assure me that you love me
Not for any talents or accomplishments,
But merely because I am one of your
Glorious creations.
Amen.

May Today There Be Peace Within

May today there be peace within.
May you trust your highest power
      that you are exactly where
      you are meant to be.
May you not forget the infinite
      possibilities that are born of faith.
May you use those gifts that you have received,
      and pass on the love that has been given to you.
May you be content knowing
      you are a child of God
Let this presence settle into your bones,
      and allow your soul the freedom to sing,
      dance, praise and love.
It is there for each and every one of you.

                    St. Thérèse of Lisieux

Chapter Five

Special Situations

*"Be strong and bold; have no fear or dread of them,
because it is the Lord your God who goes with you;
he will not fail you or forsake you."*

Deuteronomy 31:6

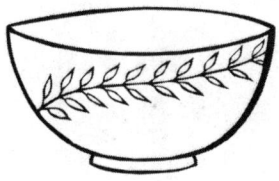

Miscarriages and Stillbirth

A miscarriage is difficult for any expectant parent. But when the miscarriage comes after we have had difficulty conceiving, or if we have had recurrent miscarriages, the pain is devastating. It seems utterly cruel to have the great hopes and dreams that come with pregnancy be followed by the emptiness of miscarriage or stillbirth. It is made even harder because, unlike other deaths, the deaths of preborn infants are not routinely acknowledged or grieved.

Experts estimate that nearly 15 percent of all pregnancies end in miscarriage, and that rate rises steadily as women age, according to the National Institute of Child Health and Human Development. In addition, 1 in nearly 200 births is a stillbirth. A couple that suffers three or more miscarriages is considered infertile and is usually referred to a specialist for testing and treatment.

As a society, we have made great strides in the past decade or so in acknowledging the loss that comes with an unfulfilled pregnancy. But we still have a long way to go. Some states require that parents be given their child's remains to bury; in other places hospitals are reluctant to surrender them, or parents don't find out about the option until it is too late. Some churches have comforting rituals available to help families in their grief, while others aren't sure what to do when the situation arises. As with infertility, family and friends try to help, but only those who have suffered this sort of loss know how devastating it is.

Grieving the loss that comes with miscarriage or stillbirth is like grieving any other death. There's no way to know what form it will take or how long it will last. Some people find comfort in returning to work as soon as possible; others need time off. Some need to cry a lot and talk about their child; others prefer meditation, prayer and silence. Many feel disoriented, or tired all the time; many also feel guilty for their child's death, no matter what the circumstances. These are all a normal part of the grieving process.

There are steps specific to miscarriage and loss that can help a grieving couple to heal. Parents often find it comforting to give their child a name. It gives them a way to remember the child in their prayers and to include it in their family history. Even if the loss is very early in pregnancy, or if the miscarriage is one of several, naming a child can give him or her an identity to match the many hopes and dreams that came with conception.

Many churches will hold a funeral or memorial service for a miscarried or stillborn child, no matter how old the child was when he or she died. There is an excerpt from a prayer service listed at the end of this chapter to help any clergyperson who might be unfamiliar with this type of service. These rituals help us to acknowledge the magnitude of the loss.

Many hospitals allow burial of remains and often work with local funeral homes or cemeteries to provide this service. In addition, some churches hold annual observances for parents to remember and honor their infants.

Secondary Infertility

When my son was two years old, we were involved in a play group that met weekly during the school year. We returned in September to greet all the friends we had missed during the summer. As we approached the playroom, I saw three mothers I had been friendly with the year before, standing in a circle talking with one another. I called out to them and all three turned around. All were visibly pregnant and radiant. I had spent the summer in fertility treatments, trying to conceive a second child, and we had just resolved to pursue adoption instead. I was happy with our decision, but seeing three friends—all with children my son's age, and all with second children on the way—reawakened feelings of frustration and inadequacy over our infertility. I smiled and chatted with them, then cried in the car the whole way home.

Infertility is different for a couple who already has one or more children. It's known as secondary infertility (as opposed to primary infertility, which describes a couple having difficulty conceiving their first child), and it's very isolating for those who experience it. We find ourselves stranded between two worlds, the fertile and the infertile, and it is difficult for us to find either sympathy for our pain or a social circle in which we feel comfortable.

We don't fit in with people who are struggling to have their first child, because secondary infertility is so different from primary infertility. We might feel guilty around couples with no children. We know those couples might resent us for wanting more. Those of us trying to conceive again might also feel ungrateful for the gift of the child (or children) we already have. In my case, I had friends who had undergone infertility treatments with me three years earlier who still hadn't conceived. Who was I to complain when they would do anything to be a parent like I already was?

But we don't fit in particularly well with the other parents we know either, who may assume that a couple with secondary infertility should be able to conceive again because we've succeeded in the past. And while the childless can avoid many situations involving children, parents with secondary infertility must be involved in our child's activities, which means being around pregnant women and babies and families who are growing exactly as we want our own family to grow.

People with secondary infertility must also grapple with what their infertility means to the child or children we already have: Isn't the child we already have enough? Why am I dissatisfied enough to want another? If we decide to seek treatment for infertility, won't we be spending money that we should be saving for our living child's education? How do I go through strenuous medical procedures with a toddler around? Does my child need a sibling? This pain is often exacerbated when the child becomes old enough to beg his or her parents for a sibling, unaware of his or her parents' struggle to do so.

Secondary infertility can bewilder couples who conceived easily in previous attempts. We might delay seeking treatment because we think that if we conceived without trouble before, we'll be able to do it again. We don't want to believe we have a problem, and we don't want to seek treatment that we believe is arduous and expensive if we don't have to. Unfortunately, the longer we wait, the less effective treatment can be if we are in our mid-thirties or older.

Parenting can be especially difficult in the midst of secondary infertility. Some parents become overly protective and worry that something may happen to the only child we have. We can put pressure on our existing child or children to fulfill all our dreams, as our dream of an additional child becomes uncertain. We can greet our

Secondary infertility can bewilder couples who conceived easily in previous attempts.

child's milestones, such as starting grade school or learning to read, with sadness because we don't know if we'll experience such moments ever again.

While some of the issues presented by secondary infertility are unique, many are the same as for any infertile couple. We envy our friends, co-workers and relatives who are welcoming new babies into their families. We sometimes have trouble communicating with one another as we search for a resolution. We worry about the costs of treatment or adoption. We struggle with the notion that we might not have the exact family we always dreamed of.

It's harder for people with secondary infertility to find others in the same situation, but not impossible. Either online or through informal networking, parents who long for another child will find it helpful to turn to others in the same situation for encouragement and solace. Sharing this particular sorrow doesn't make it go away, but it helps to lessen the burden to know that we are not alone.

Infertility and Step-Parenting

To outsiders, step-parenting while trying to have a child might seem like a fortunate turn of events. Aspiring parents get to practice their cuddling and disciplinary skills as they wait to conceive, and the happy chaos of having children around helps fill the time they'd otherwise spend pining for children of their own.

The reality, though, is often far different. Step-parenting is difficult and sometimes lonely work. Infertility is physically and emotionally draining. Taken together, the challenges of step-parenting while trying to conceive can overwhelm. Step-parents often find that being involved in their step-children's lives seems harder than enduring infertility alone as a couple.

Much of this has to do with the difficult nature of step-parenting in general. Especially early in a marriage, step-parents struggle to find their role and to gain acceptance from the children of their new spouse. It can take years for a new step-parent to find a comfortable way of relating to and being involved in their step-children's lives.

This delicate relationship takes on new complexity if a couple runs into trouble conceiving. Like those with secondary infertility, step-parents are forced to be around children, even when doing so is painful or upsetting. Even the fun things step-parents do with step-children—reading bedtime stories, going on vacation, attending soccer games—are reminders of all the things they want to do with their own children and of the fear they never will. The blessings of parenthood, when one longs to be a parent, can feel like salt in a wound.

In some ways, being a step-parent means enduring the pain of infertility alone, because he or she is married to someone who is already a parent. Yes, a couple goes through infertility together, but something changes when one of them already has children. They have experienced the thrill of doctor's appointments and the excitement of coming home from the hospital. They know what it's like to be up all night with a sick child or to see their baby walk for the first time. And so, no matter how supportive or compassionate a spouse is, those without children can feel isolated.

There is no easy solution to the difficulties faced by infertile step-parents. But perhaps it helps to remember that, even though the circumstances of step-parenting can make infertility more painful, in the end they are two separate things, and each deserves its own appropriate response. Infertility makes physical, emotional and financial demands on us, and step-children have their own demands on time and emotions. But children deserve and require love and attention from the adults in their lives. It's up to the adults—parents and step-parents alike—to do everything they can to make sure the children receive it.

PRAYER AND REFLECTION

John 14:1-4

"Do not let your hearts be troubled. Believe in God, believe also in me. In my Father's house there are many dwelling-places. If it were not so, would I have told you that I go to prepare a place for you? And if I go and prepare a place for you, I will come again and will take you to myself, so that where I am there you may be also. And you know the way to the place where I am going."

Prayer of St. Augustine

God of our life, there are days when the burdens we carry chafe our shoulders and weigh us down; when the road seems dreary and endless, the skies grey and threatening; when our lives have no music in them, and our hearts are lonely, and our souls have lost their courage. Flood the path with light, run our eyes to where the skies are full of promise; tune our hearts to brave music; give us the sense of comradeship with heroes and saints of every age; and so quicken our spirits that we may be able to encourage the souls of all who journey with us on the road of life, to your honor and glory.

Serenity Prayer
Attributed to Reinhold Niebuhr

God grant me the serenity
to accept the things I cannot change;
courage to change the things I can;
and wisdom to know the difference.

Living one day at a time;
enjoying one moment at a time;
accepting hardships as the pathway to peace;
taking, as he did, this sinful world
as it is, not as I would have it;
trusting that he will make all things right
if I surrender to his will;
that I may be reasonably happy in this life
and supremely happy with him
forever in the next.
Amen.

Father and Creator, in whom all life and death find their meaning, we bless you at all times, especially when we stand in need of your comfort.

We entrust to your care a life conceived in love. May your blessing now come upon us. Remove from us all anxiety of mind, Strengthen this love so that we may have peace in our hearts and in our home.

We ask this in the Name of Christ, Our Lord, your Only-begotten Son, who said to us that anything we asked in his name would be given us.

A Blessing of Parents after a Miscarriage

Chapter Six

Making Decisions

Do not worry about anything,
but in everything by prayer and supplication
with thanksgiving let your requests be made known to God.
And the peace of God, which surpasses all understanding,
will guard your hearts and your minds in Christ Jesus.

Philippians 4:6-7

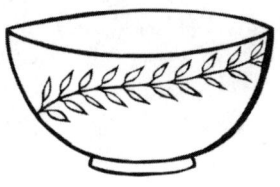

WHEN I FIRST BEGAN TO WORRY that my husband and I might be infertile, I made an appointment with a gynecologist. As I sat in his office he explained the diagnostic tests he would run and mentioned possible treatments, including in-vitro fertilization.

"We're not interested in that," I said quickly, explaining that my husband and I had already decided it was too drastic and went against the teachings of the Catholic Church.

"Well that's good," he replied, "because it's very expensive and it rarely works."

A year later we sat in the office of a reproductive endocrinologist who explained that, after several failed intra-uterine inseminations, in-vitro was our only option.

"When can we begin?" I asked, eager to start the treatment I'd flatly dismissed only a year ago. (When in-vitro finally led to the birth of our son, I thought about sending a picture of him to the first gynecologist, along with a suggestion that he choose his words more carefully in the future, but I never quite got around to it.)

I'm not proud that, faced with dwindling options, my principles changed so drastically in such a short time. But I'm not ashamed either. Our decision to pursue in-vitro fertilization was the culmination of a long process of discernment that included talking to three priests, reading the Catechism of the Catholic Church, praying, and discussing our future at great length. Even after we changed our minds about in-vitro, we still decided that we weren't comfortable with donor eggs or sperm, nor would we discard excess embryos. The process taught me the importance of having principles to guide us, and the importance of being flexible enough to consider other options when the territory around us changes.

The following two chapters examine the specific decisions we face in treatment and beyond treatment. In this chapter, the focus is on thinking about how and why we decide which path to pursue. Infertility very quickly becomes an exhausting and seemingly endless series of decisions. How long should we wait before seeking medical help? Do we start off with a gynecologist or go straight to a fertility specialist? What sorts of treatments are we willing to pursue? Would we consider IVF, freezing embryos, donor sperm, or eggs? Should we look into adoption? What about remaining childless?

Just as there is no one right way to become a parent, there is no best approach to deciding how to tackle infertility. It will be different for each couple, and each person. By taking some time to figure out how to best arrive at difficult decisions, and by making time to pray for discernment and guidance, we can make an arduous process a little easier on ourselves.

Researching the Options

Perhaps it's just my nature, but I found it helpful to begin by learning everything I could about our options. I liked knowing that our intra-uterine inseminations had a 20 percent chance of working, and that adoptions qualify for a $10,000 federal tax credit. Knowledge helped me understand what we faced, and it helped me explain our options to my husband, who's not quite so research-oriented.

Knowledge also makes us effective partners in our medical treatment. No matter how good our doctors may be, they can't make our decisions for us. A 5 percent chance of conception may be acceptable odds for one couple and unacceptable for another; $20,000 in doctors' fees is negligible for some but out of the question for many. Knowing beforehand the odds and the costs of treatment allows us to actively decide which path to pursue rather than passively follow a treatment path that we may later come to regret.

For those who find power in knowledge, there is almost an inexhaustible source of information online and at bookstores. Many books and web sites are available to educate patients about infertility, so we may become informed consumers of medical treatment. Not every resource is reliable, but at the very least reading and learning about infertility arms patients with questions we need to ask our doctors.

Not everyone, of course, wants or needs to know the range of acceptable day-3 FSH numbers, or the possible benefits of replacing low-fat dairy with high-fat dairy while trying to conceive. For many it's too exhausting and overwhelming to research every possible aspect of infertility. And there are doctors who wish the Internet would simply go away, because many patients equate a few hours online with a degree in reproductive endocrinology. The first specialist we saw made me promise to stop looking at web sites after I told him my post-ovulatory progesterone levels showed my luteal phase was of sufficient length. And to an extent he was right: He was the doctor. If his references and our comfort level with him were good, I needed to sit back and trust him to treat us.

Every time an option fails we think there must be another line of treatment to pursue, another specialist to consult.

So whether we're just beginning to look into treatment or we are infertility veterans, it's worth thinking and talking about how much we want to participate in our treatment. Start by checking a book out of the library and looking through it. By the end it will probably be clear whether you want to know more or whether that's quite enough.

Setting Limits

We are fortunate to live in a time when so many options exist for infertile couples. Every year thousands of people become biological parents who wouldn't have had a chance of doing so even ten years ago. Every year it seems that doctors find new techniques that extend the promise of parenthood to even more people.

But those options can be dangerously seductive, because every time an option fails we think there must be another line of treatment to pursue, another specialist to consult. People travel all over the country, and sometimes all over the world, seeking a new technique that holds the promise of pregnancy. The promise often comes at great price. And whether the cost is financial, physical or emotional, it's hard to say no to something we want so badly.

That is why it's smart for couples to talk, realistically and openly, about the limits of what we are willing to do to conceive. Pursuing pregnancy without an end in mind can be devastating to marriages, bank accounts, and mental health. By setting limits, even if we give ourselves the flexibility to change our minds at a later date, we are less likely to continue pursuing treatment that we will later regret.

Given that high-tech infertility treatments are often not covered by health insurance, many couples encounter financial limits first. How much are we willing to spend on medical treatment? What is an adequate trade-off when it comes to chances of success versus cost? Is it worth spending $15,000 on an IVF cycle that has only a 10 percent chance of working? If adoption is an alternative, will another IVF cycle jeopardize our chances of paying for adoption?

Finances aren't the only consideration. Infertility treatment can be physically grueling and, while the research is not conclusive, there is the possibility that it increases our chances of some health problems in the future. Any woman who is considering taking fertility drugs should consult her doctor about the possible long-term health risks involved.

How will we know when our bodies have had enough? Some couples find it helpful to set limits based on time, such as, we'll try this for a year and evaluate our choices at the end of that year. For others, it is the unpredictability of treatment and its emotional costs that help us know when we need to pursue another option. Men and women tend to set limits differently, with men more concerned about finances and women assuming an "anything it takes" attitude. The limits are different for every couple facing infertility, but it's important for every one of them to examine their options and set limits away from the pressures of the doctor's office. Doing so increases the chances that we will make decisions we can live with for the rest of our lives.

Time Off for Discernment

Taking a break from our attempts at parenthood is another essential part of the decision-making process. If we are single-minded about conceiving, even a month off can feel like a missed opportunity and a waste of time. When we've been waiting so long, and organizing our lives around our wish to conceive, the thought of even a few extra weeks is excruciating. We think, what if this was the month it was meant to be? But just as our bodies need rest on a regular basis, our minds need time to unwind and focus on other things. These periods of rest and reflection give us time to consider other opportunities. We may find our minds drifting or settling on new options if we give them the time and space to wander rather than remaining fixed on one goal.

In times of treatment and during time off, prayer and meditation are important to the process of discernment.

Perhaps it's a few minutes every day spent in quiet reflection, or a Rosary recited as we fall asleep. Maybe it's enough to arrive for Sunday services a few minutes early, or it's enough to stay late and devote that time to praying for God's guidance on our journey. Some churches offer support groups for people trying to conceive; these offer a welcome chance to meet with others who are facing the same challenges and can offer new ways of approaching infertility. A retreat, alone or with our spouse, can be a welcome chance to consider our options away from the demands of daily life.

In this hectic and emotional time, we need to listen to God and consider what God might be telling us, rather than always telling God what we need and want. The best way to ensure that we actually do this is to set time aside and devote it solely to praying for guidance. There is enormous pressure to act, and the infertile usually want our ordeal over with as quickly as possible. But momentous decisions deserve our careful deliberation and prayer.

PRAYER AND REFLECTION

Romans 8:26-28
Likewise the Spirit helps us in our weakness; for we do not know how to pray as we ought, but that very Spirit intercedes with sighs too deep for words. And God, who searches the heart, knows what is the mind of the Spirit, because the Spirit intercedes for the saints according to the will of God.

Prayer for Discernment

By Thomas Merton

My Lord God, I have no idea where I am going.
I do not see the road ahead of me.
Nor do I really know myself.
And the fact that I think I am following your will
Does not mean that I am actually doing so.

But I believe that the desire to please you
Does in fact please you.
And I hope that I will never do anything apart from
    that desire.
And I know that if I do this,
You will lead me by the right road
Though I may know nothing about it.

Therefore I will trust you always
Though I may seem to be lost
    and in the shadow of death
I will not fear for you are ever with me.
And you will never leave me to face my struggles alone.

A Plea for Guidance

Dear God,
I am overwhelmed sometimes
With the decisions I must make
And all their possible consequences.
How can I possibly know what to do?

Yet I know what I need to do:
To slow down and remain alert,
To sit in silence and wait
For the still, small voice that will guide me
Toward the path you want me on.

And so I will listen.
All I ask is that you speak to me.
Amen.

Show Me the Course

Steer the ship of my life, good Lord, to your quiet harbor, where I can be safe from the storms of sin and conflict. Show me the course I should take. Renew in me the gift of discernment, so that I can always see the right direction in which I should go. And give me the strength and the courage to choose the right course, even when the sea is rough and the waves are high, knowing that through enduring hardship and danger in your name we shall find comfort and peace.

Basil of Caesarea (c. 329-379)

Chapter Seven

The Morality of Treatment

*You must therefore be careful to do
as the Lord your God has commanded you;
you shall not turn to the right or to the left.*

Deuteronomy 5:32

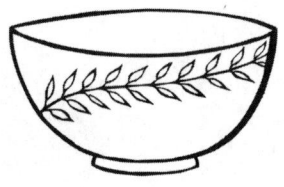

IT IS ASTONISHING to consider the advances the world has made in treating infertility over the past few decades. Doctors can now remove an egg from a woman's ovary, place it in a Petri dish, and inject a single sperm into it to bring about conception. A few days later they can take the resulting eight-celled embryo, invisible to the human eye, remove a cell, and test it for a long list of diseases. Women without uteruses can raise their own genetic offspring thanks to the use of surrogate mothers. Women who have gone through menopause and men who produce no sperm at all can use donor eggs and sperm to conceive and carry a child. Every year brings new discoveries that make biological parenthood a reality for more and more people.

But with these advances come ethical, legal and moral dilemmas that would have been unimaginable a generation ago. Surrogate mothers sometimes change their minds and fight to keep the children they've carried in their wombs. In-vitro fertilization often leaves couples with leftover embryos even after they've completed their families. Parents must decide whether to tell their children that their genetic mother or father is an anonymous donor. With every new technology comes the risk of misuse and abuse.

These issues force us to consider whether we should embrace a technology simply because it exists. At what point do children become a commodity rather than a gift from God? Do we have an absolute right to bear children, and are we allowed to use any means necessary to achieve pregnancy? Does the high cost of infertility treatment, at a time when people around the world routinely die of preventable disease, make such treatment immoral? What about the morality of insurance policies that make fertility treatment available to the rich but impossible for the poor?

Christian churches have struggled with these issues, especially since the birth of the first in-vitro baby in 1978. Obviously Jesus said nothing about this technology, but theologians use Christian principles to decide what is morally acceptable... and what is not. There is a wide range of opinions on which technologies are permissible. Some communities, such as the Baptists, tend to stress that these decisions are ultimately between individuals and God, while denominations like the Catholic Church have a centralized authority and an expectation that members will follow its teachings (though even among Catholics a well-informed conscience is the ultimate arbiter). Some churches teach that only technology using genetic material from the husband and wife is acceptable, while a few permit the involvement of other people as donors. We will look at the most common techniques below, along with the teachings from major denominations on each technique.

But first, it's important to consider not only the

We owe it to our faith to make an effort to understand the teaching and the concerns behind it.

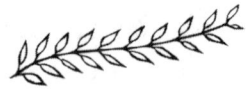

teachings of our spiritual leaders but also what we can and should do with those teachings. We live in an age when many people have a knee-jerk reaction to being told what we can and cannot do. Especially with the technology available, it can be difficult to hear that our faith forbids us from using it. I would urge anyone contemplating reproductive technology to seek to understand what their faith teaches and why. These views represent the thinking of informed and sincere followers of Christ who have reflected on and debated these medical advances at length. Even if ultimately we disagree with the teaching, we owe it to our faith to make an effort to understand the teaching and the concerns behind it.

Fertility Medications

Fertility medications are often given in pill form or by injection to help a woman ovulate or to regulate her cycle. The greatest risk comes from the fact that women usually produce more than one egg while taking these medications. This increases the possibility of conceiving twins, triplets or more. Most cases of quadruplets, quintuplets, and larger sets of births stem from the use of fertility drugs rather than in-vitro fertilization. Doctors using in-vitro are able to limit the number of fertilized eggs placed back in a woman's uterus, while they aren't able to control the number of eggs fertilized in a woman who is using fertility medication alone. Also, many women are reluctant to cancel a medicated cycle that produces a large number of eggs, even if faced with the risk of conceiving several embryos, because of the cost and time involved in taking fertility medications.

If a woman is carrying three or more fetuses, doctors may recommend that one or more be terminated, a procedure known as "selective reduction." This procedure increases the chances that the remaining fetuses will be born healthy. It can also lead to an agonizing decision for the couple involved: Abort one or more fetuses to increase the chances that one or two will survive, or continue with the pregnancy intact and risk losing them all.

In general, most Christian churches endorse the use of fertility medications without reservation. However, many Christians, including the Catholic Church and most Baptist denominations, oppose selective reduction because it is a form of abortion. Even mainline denominations that allow for abortion in some cases discourage parents from treatment that might make selective reduction medically advisable. As long as patients use fertility medications, conceiving several fetuses will always be a risk, but doctors and patients can work together to reduce the risk by closely monitoring cycles and canceling cycles that produce large numbers of eggs.

Artificial Insemination Using the Husband's Sperm

When doctors administer fertility medications to a woman, they can advise a couple to have intercourse at assigned times, or they can use assisted (or artificial) insemination around the time the woman is ovulating to further boost chances of conception. To perform assisted insemination, a man must masturbate and collect his semen in a cup. The semen is then treated and placed in a catheter that is injected into a woman's uterus. This increases the chances of conception by eliminating the need for the sperm to travel from the woman's cervix to her uterus. Artificial insemination is also used sometimes if the woman's cervical mucus is hostile to sperm, or if doctors can't determine what is preventing a couple from conceiving.

Most denominations condone the use of assisted insemination if the husband's sperm is used. The major exception to this is the Catholic Church, which opposes assisted insemination. In Catholic teaching, conception should not take place outside of intercourse, and any technique that bypasses lovemaking makes conception immoral. The Catholic Church, along with a few other denominations, opposes the use of masturbation to collect the semen. Couples who wish to avoid masturbation can collect sperm by using a condom during intercourse (some theologians advise the condom have tiny holes in it, to allow for at least a theoretical chance of natural conception). One drawback to this, from a medical perspective, is that perforating the condom can lower the amount of semen collected.

Artificial Insemination Using Donor Sperm

If a man's sperm count is very low, or if a couple has tried artificial insemination without success, one possible option is to use assisted insemination with a donor's sperm. In the past it was up to doctors to select the donor, but now prospective parents can look at profiles of donors to select someone based on compatible physical traits, professional interests, or athletic ability. Assisted insemination using a donor's sperm is also an option for single women or female same-sex couples who wish to become pregnant. The insemination proceeds as described above, with the sperm injected into the woman's uterus. The woman is usually on fertility medications so doctors can control when she will ovulate, thereby timing the insemination to achieve the greatest chances of success.

The identity of donors was once a tightly-guarded secret, and many parents never told their children that they were conceived using donor sperm. But it is becoming more common for donors and prospective parents alike to at least consider the possibility that children could someday contact their biological fathers. As we learn more about the genetic causes of disease, more and more parents are finding it important for their children to know their medical background, which requires telling them the details of their conception.

In general, most Christian churches disapprove of using donor sperm for artificial insemination, and even some fairly-liberal denominations find the practice controversial. Because it involves the genetic material of someone outside the marriage, some theologians liken donor insemination to adultery. They worry about the long-term effects on a marriage and family when the mother is genetically related to their children and the father is not. There is also concern for the confusion that children might feel when they learn that they were conceived via donor insemination and for the burden of secrecy if the family decides not to share the details with outsiders.

In the 1990s doctors began using a technique that, in many cases, has eliminated the need for donor sperm. Known as intro-cytoplasmic sperm injection (ICSI), doctors use it as part of a cycle of in-vitro fertilization when there are doubts about a man's sperm count or quality. ICSI allows most men a chance at genetic fatherhood, even those who previously would have had little hope of conceiving. However, ICSI makes already-expensive IVF cycles even more expensive, and there are still some men for whom ICSI is not an option.

In-Vitro Fertilization Using the Wife's Eggs
When it was first successfully used in 1978, in-vitro fertilization seemed like something out of a science-fiction novel, with eggs and sperm united under the bright lights of a laboratory instead of mysteriously in a woman's womb. Now IVF is almost commonplace. Most people know at least one couple who has used IVF to conceive, and the technique has directly led to the births of hundreds of thousands of babies worldwide. While there have been some advancements, the basics of IVF remain the same. Doctors administer fertility drugs to the woman, enabling her to produce many eggs instead of the one per month that most women produce. When the eggs are ready, the doctor removes them from the woman, and they are placed in a Petri dish along with her

husband's sperm (or doctors inject sperm directly into the egg, the technique known as ICSI explained above). After waiting a few days to see which eggs fertilize and which resulting embryos continue growing, doctors choose a few embryos to return to the woman's uterus. Any leftover embryos are frozen for future IVF cycles. A pregnancy test two weeks later determines if the cycle has worked.

Most Christian churches approve the use of IVF as long as the eggs and sperm derive from the couple who wish to become parents. The teachings of the Roman Catholic Church oppose IVF, even when the spouses' sperm and eggs are used. Catholics oppose IVF because conception takes place outside the act of lovemaking and outside the body, and because it requires the involvement of people outside the marriage. Catholic leaders are also concerned about the fate of unused embryos which are either frozen or, ultimately, discarded. The Eastern Orthodox Church discourages IVF because of the large number of embryos that die, either after being transferred back to the woman's uterus or as a result of freezing. Christian Scientists also generally oppose in-vitro fertilization because of the advanced medical technology required to bring about conception.

The practice of freezing leftover embryos and the question of what to do with unwanted embryos are important ethical considerations for any couple thinking about using IVF. When a medical office freezes leftover embryos, it is unlikely that they will all survive the process of thawing. Some people rationalize the decision by saying that any embryo that can't survive being frozen and then thawed probably wouldn't survive long enough to implant itself in a woman's womb. But for people who believe that life begins at the moment of conception, deciding to freeze an embryo that might not make it through the thawing process can be viewed as the murder of a child. Prospective parents who aren't comfortable with the idea of freezing can choose to fertilize only as many eggs as they can return to the woman's womb, although limiting the number of fertilized eggs does lower the chance for success. This is a matter of utmost moral gravity that a couple should decide long before they reach the stage of retrieving the woman's eggs.

The issue of unwanted embryos has been in the news for years, linked to the issue of stem-cell research. By most estimates there are hundreds of thousands of such embryos sitting in storage in fertility clinics all over the United States. It is difficult for many couples to imagine a situation in which we would have more embryos than we could want, because we have likely suffered many disappointments in our attempts to conceive and we fear we never will. But for many, it is a very real possibility. Couples who choose IVF must decide in advance what we will do if our efforts succeed beyond our expectations.

Most clinics give patients the option of thawing the embryos, donating them for research, donating them to another couple, or transferring them to a woman's uterus at a time in her cycle when conception is impossible. All of these options have advantages and disadvantages, depending on a couple's beliefs and wishes. Thawing the embryos and disposing of them is perhaps the quickest and most common resolution, but for those who believe the embryos are living or even potential human beings, throwing them away might seem cruel and immoral. Donating the embryos to research could provide important clues in the treatment of disease, but such research nearly always requires destruction of the organisms. So for people who view embryos as a form of life, this too is a method of murder. Donating embryos to another couple—known as "embryo adoption"—is a way for couples who have completed their families to ensure the embryos have a shot at survival. However, some people are uncomfortable with the idea of having their genetic offspring raised in another family. Finally, transferring the embryos back to the woman's uterus when conception is unlikely, which is known as a "compassionate transfer," is reassuring for some people because the embryos expire inside the woman's body. But again, a couple who believes the embryos are living beings might be troubled by this practice because the embryos have no realistic chance of survival.

In-Vitro Fertilization Using Donor Eggs

When a woman doesn't ovulate, or when her eggs are of poor quality, or when her attempts at IVF have failed repeatedly, she may still become pregnant using donated eggs. Doctors give hormones to the donor, retrieve eggs from her, fertilize those eggs with the sperm from the prospective father, then transfer the resulting embryos into the uterus of the prospective mother.

Couples who choose to use donor eggs appreciate that the woman is able to experience pregnancy and childbirth. The technique also allows prospective parents to provide good prenatal care and avoid exposure to drugs, alcohol, and other possible harm. In addition, many people are also comforted that at least one parent — the father — is genetically related to the child.

Most Christian churches, however, oppose IVF with donor eggs for the same reasons they oppose donor sperm. They believe that conception achieved with eggs from a woman outside the marriage is akin to adultery. This can create tension within a marriage, especially if the parents choose not to tell others about

Couples who choose to use donor eggs appreciate that the woman is able to experience pregnancy and childbirth.

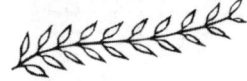

how their children were conceived. There are the same issues of possible identity confusion and anger among children when they learn of their origins, although many families who use donor eggs share the information early with their children and treat it as a form of adoption.

Egg donation is a much more involved process than sperm donation. The role of the egg donor must be carefully considered as well. Medical practices and private brokers recruit young women to donate their eggs, and most screen them carefully to rule out both inherited disease and psychological instability. The process requires donors to inject themselves with hormones, undergo minor surgery, and be available for frequent doctor's appointments for up to one month.

In other countries, egg donors have their medical care covered but aren't allowed any payment for their eggs. In the U.S., the market is unregulated, and donors are routinely paid for their eggs — anywhere from $5,000 up to many tens of thousands of dollars, if a donor meets certain requirements that a couple is looking for (for example, if she attends a prestigious college, has exemplary SAT scores, or meets height or weight requirements). Most donors report that they are motivated by a mix of altruism and the desire for money.

It is troubling to think that a couple would pay $100,000 for the eggs of a 5' 10" volleyball player from Stanford who scored 1600 on her SATs, and such a practice clearly views a child as a commodity rather than a blessing and a miracle. But those cases remain rare. Most couples who use donor eggs simply want someone who resembles the intended mother enough that a resulting child might look like the woman who will raise him or her. Still, because the market for egg donations is not regulated, unscrupulous brokers exist who can take advantage of desperate couples. Anyone contemplating the use of donor eggs should pick a medical practice carefully and read more about the legal and psychological aspects of egg donation. We should also explore with one another and in prayer why we want to use donor eggs, whom we will tell about our decision, and what we will tell our child about his or her origins.

Surrogacy

The practice of surrogacy dates to at least Biblical times and the story of Abraham, Sarah and Hagar. Records indicate it was a common practice in ancient times. More recently, many people remember the 1986 saga of Baby M, the infant girl whose surrogate mother, Mary Beth Whitehead, refused to surrender her after giving birth. Mrs. Whitehead had been hired by William Stern, the baby's biological father, and his wife to act as a surrogate. Mrs. Whitehead eventually lost her battle to keep custody of the baby, and the case led to a tightening in the laws surrounding surrogacy to ensure that surrogates fulfill the terms of the contracts they sign.

There are two forms of surrogacy: traditional surrogacy, in which the surrogate becomes pregnant using her own eggs and the intended father's sperm, either through insemination or IVF, and gestational surrogacy, in which the mother's eggs or the eggs of a donor are fertilized with her husband's sperm and the resulting embryos are transferred to the surrogate, who carries the pregnancy to term and delivers the child. Using a donor's eggs has become more common since the Baby M case because it avoids the possible difficulty a surrogate might have surrendering her own genetic child. In traditional surrogacy the child is genetically related to the surrogate; in gestational surrogacy the child is genetically related to the mother or the donor, rather than the surrogate.

Most Christian traditions object to traditional surrogacy on the same grounds that they oppose egg donation: They teach that the involvement of a third party for reproduction violates the sanctity of a marriage. This is even more pronounced in surrogacy than in egg donation. Couples who use donor eggs usually never meet the donor, and her involvement ends even before conception. But a surrogate's involvement lasts for nine months, and often beyond. In most cases the couple and the surrogate are well-equipped to handle any strain, and there are many examples of couples who forge close, long-lasting relationships with their surrogates. Nevertheless, couples should be aware that the involvement of a third person in reproduction, and especially the high level of involvement created by surrogacy, can create strain on a marriage in unexpected ways and for many years to come.

Religious thinkers express concern for the effect that surrogacy has on children, especially those produced from traditional surrogacy, in which their birth mothers conceived and carried them knowing they would not raise them. Again, in most cases children borne of surrogacy are happy and well-adjusted, but in some cases the circumstances of their births create confusion or anger. Couples who are considering a surrogacy arrangement must talk openly about how they will explain it to their children and how they will face problems that arise from it.

Finally, it is important to consider the surrogate mother and the effects the arrangement might have on her. Some theologians and feminists argue that surrogacy can exploit younger, poorer women hired to carry pregnancies for women who are usually older and wealthier, because surrogates are often paid for the service. While it's true that few women would choose to be a surrogate simply to make money, and most describe a sense of satisfaction from helping a couple become parents, surrogacy is a very complicated relationship that can engender unexpected feelings of regret and confusion. Most surrogates undergo psychological screening to ensure they will be able to fulfill their role without second guesses, but couples thinking about surrogacy also need to consider what the effects of the arrangement might be on the surrogate and whether they are comfortable with the possible implications.

Surrogacy is a very complicated relationship that can engender unexpected feelings of regret and confusion.

Many people argue that third-party reproduction is similar to adoption in that a child's biological parent(s) differ from the parents who raise the child. But in most adoptions, the pregnancy is unplanned, and adoption provides a loving family to a child who already exists. In third-party reproduction, a child is created with the knowledge that at least one of its genetic parents will not raise it. This prior knowledge is troubling to many religious thinkers and sets third-party reproduction apart from adoption.

One can be a good Christian and still choose, after careful deliberation and prayer, to use the high-tech treatments discussed in this chapter. I have attempted to explain the sometimes-controversial positions of many Christian traditions. Even if a couple concludes that we disagree with our faith's position on a technique, it is a valuable exercise to understand the position and the arguments behind it. It is essential for couples to talk over these issues and decide how our values will influence our decisions before we begin fertility treatment. To do any less is unfair to ourselves and any children we might create.

PRAYER AND REFLECTION

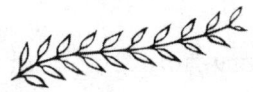

Philippians 1:9-11
And this is my prayer: that your love may overflow more and more with knowledge and full insight to help you to determine what is best, so that on the day of Christ you may be pure and blameless, having produced the harvest of righteousness that comes through Jesus Christ for the glory and the praise of God.

Prayer for God's Guidance
By St. Teresa of Avila

Govern everything by your wisdom, O Lord,
so that my soul may always be serving you
in the way you will
and not as I choose.
Let me die to myself so that I may serve you;
let me live to you who are life itself.
Amen.

O Lord, Help Me Decide

O Lord,
I am astonished sometimes
When I think of everything that man can do:
Fly to the outer reaches of your earth,
Bring back the living from near death,
Create a baby where once there was no hope.
We thank you for these technological advances.
And we ask for your help in navigating
The difficult decisions that sometimes
accompany them.
O Lord, help me decide what is of you and from you
And give me the courage to follow your guidance,
Especially when it's so hard to do so.
We ask this in Jesus' name.
Amen.

Prayer of John Henry Newman

I will trust Him. Whatever, wherever I am, I can never be thrown away. If I am in sickness, my sickness may serve Him; in perplexity, my perplexity may serve Him; if I am in sorrow, my sorrow may serve Him. My sickness, or perplexity, or sorrow may be necessary causes of some great end, which is quite beyond us. He does nothing in vain.

Chapter Eight

Moving On

Be still before the Lord; and wait patiently for him;
do not fret over those who prosper in their way,
over those who carry out evil devices.

Psalm 37:7

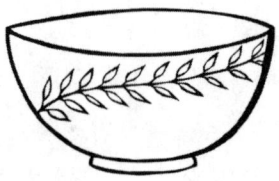

THE DECISION TO STOP THE PURSUIT of biological parenthood comes at a different time for everyone. I know people who have spent more than a decade—and incredible sums of money—pursuing treatment around the globe. I also know of a couple who, after six months of attempting to conceive, went to a gynecologist who explained the tests they could run. The couple rejected it all outright and began adoption work right away. Everyone is different, and we all approach the timing and details of such a decision in different ways.

Of course, the cessation of treatment doesn't rule out pregnancy entirely. We've all heard stories of "miracle babies" conceived after their parents had given up. But sometimes holding out for a miracle prevents us from pursuing other options, such as adoption or foster parenting, or even from taking a new job that we're afraid might interfere with a pregnancy. There is nothing wrong with continuing to pray for conception even after it seems unlikely. But it is exhausting to plan our lives around the idea that we may become pregnant next month, or the month after. If it seems very unlikely, then at some point it helps to make a decision to move on.

It's best, in the days and weeks following a decision to stop treatment, not to rush into anything else. Our bodies, minds and souls need time to recuperate, and to absorb new ways of imagining our futures. It is best at this moment to live instinctively—to cry whenever it feels necessary, to sleep a lot or eat chocolate or take a fabulous cruise to Mexico. Perhaps the most important thing a couple can do is to share our pain with one another and not allow the loss to come between us.

Grieving the Loss of Fertility

Couples who decide, or who are told by a doctor, that fertility treatment is no longer an option, need time to grieve. It's likely we've assumed since childhood that we will bear children someday, and when we realize we probably never will, it is absolutely a form of death. Even if our options have looked increasingly grim, it is still quite a blow to finally admit that biological parenthood is extremely unlikely or impossible. We must surrender the dream of a child who looks like us. We must give up a biological connection, not only to a child but also to our spouse through conceiving a child. Often we fear disappointing our own parents, who also will likely grieve the loss of a biological grandchild.

Like all grief, it is impossible to tell how long it will take to recover from this particular loss or what exactly will help. Our struggles with infertility are often hidden from public view, and so when we surrender in our quest to conceive a child, it too often takes place in private. But just as the public ritual of a funeral helps mourners understand and accept their loss, so too can a ritual help close this chapter of our lives. A sympathetic clergy member can likely suggest or develop a ceremony to commemorate this moment. Or a couple may prefer to create a ritual of their own—a short prayer, a reading from Scripture, even a moment of silence in which they ask for God's help to navigate the future.

While most people grieve the realization that they will likely never conceive, some also experience relief. Actively pursuing pregnancy is exhausting. It controls our time, our finances, our minds, and our emotions. When we stop, our lives are ours again. We can schedule trips out of town without worry of interfering with treatment schedules. We can make love with our spouse whenever we feel like it, instead of having a doctor dictate when and how often. We are free to pursue the pastimes and relationships that may have suffered in our all-consuming efforts. There is nothing wrong with feeling relief that this time in our lives is over. It doesn't mean that we never really wanted to conceive; it means that we are justly pleased to be free of the constraints that infertility has placed on our lives.

There is nothing wrong with feeling relief that this time in our lives is over.

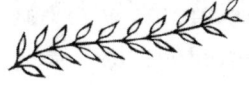

Conversely, some people find they miss the excitement and hope that fertility treatments represent, even if those hopes are routinely dashed. Doctors' appointments and medications provide a schedule and a structure to our lives, and there is always the dangling possibility that our efforts may pay off. When we stop this active pursuit, we might find ourselves feeling unmoored and bereft. Something that has likely assumed a central place in our lives, perhaps for years, is now suddenly gone. Some of us might feel strange. We miss the grueling schedule of treatments and even the discomfort of examinations and shots. But this too is a perfectly normal reaction to the stress we've been living in. It takes some time to adjust to life beyond fertility treatment, and it may require us to think of ourselves in a new way.

Telling Others

It is comforting at this time to find other people who have moved on from their pursuit of pregnancy, if only to see that it is possible to find joy even if our deepest wishes remain unfulfilled. Couples who are interested in adoption can easily find parents who decided to adopt after attempting to conceive. It is also helpful to talk with couples who have chosen not to have children and have instead invested their energy in careers, volunteer work, and relationships. These families are invaluable resources as we begin our journey forward. God places these people in our lives so that we don't have to carry on all alone.

Like others who are grieving, we may hear well-meaning but hurtful comments from other people when we tell them that we likely won't be conceiving. Many will offer unwanted advice or share an anecdote about couples who decided to adopt and got pregnant the next month. It is best to practice tactful silence when these moments arrive, or come up with a short, standard answer that cuts off the conversation.

Some people may raise the idea that not everyone is meant to have children, and that children are a gift from God. This can sound to the infertile couple as though God is punishing them by not bestowing the gift of children. Whenever I heard someone say this, it always sounded to me like children are a reward for good behavior, which of course isn't true.

I suppose it's normal, when people are faced with a difficult situation like a friend's infertility, to try to come up with a simple explanation for it. The truth is there is no simple way to understand why some people are unable to conceive. It is possible that those for whom medical treatment fails are being called to do something else; it may remain a mystery, and a gaping wound, for the rest of their lives. But no one will be able to adequately explain to a grieving couple why they cannot bear children. That answer is for God alone to reveal.

As they begin to heal, there will come a time when it feels right to start thinking about other options. This is a moment when they profoundly need to listen to God in prayer, as God will help move them from disappointment to a new beginning. Many couples who have tried without success to conceive begin by thinking of anything else as Plan B. They have their hearts set on conception and they view other paths, whether adoption or living childfree, as second-best. Quiet, committed prayer can help move them from ambivalence to excitement, from the heartbreak of infertility to a joy that can unfold in surprising ways. It seems especially important to emphasize listening in prayer at this time, because by turning their attention to God, they allow God the time and space to address their fears and answer their pleas.

PRAYER AND REFLECTION

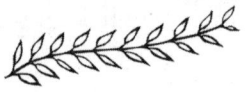

Psalm 71: 20-21
You who have made me see many troubles and calamities will revive me again; from the depths of the earth you will bring me up again. You will increase my honor, and comfort me once again.

Psalm 34:17-20
When the righteous cry for help, the Lord hears, and rescues them from all their troubles. The Lord is near to the brokenhearted, and saves the crushed in spirit. Many are the afflictions of the righteous, but the Lord rescues them from them all.

A Prayer to a Listening God

By John McCullough Bade

O God, we labor in the heat of the day,
     and so often the labor feels hopeless,
     unproductive, useless ....

And yet, you hear our silent cries.
You give us one another
     to speak that which we in our pain cannot speak.
You give us your Word
     that utters those things we cannot find
     the words to say.

And not only do you give us the words to speak,
     but you also turn your ear to us and hear us,
     even when all we have strength to whisper is,
       "Lord, in your mercy, hear our prayer."

For you have promised to hear us.
You have promised to turn your face to shine upon us.
You have promised to be our shade
     when the heat of the day saps our strength
     and the well of hope runs dry.

And you have promised,
     even in the silence,
       to give us the sweet sound of peace.

For Strength

Dear Lord,
I am crushed.
I've always hoped and prayed for a different answer.
This "no" echoes in my bones,
Sends anguish into the deepest part of my soul.

I can ask for nothing else than your tender care
In this time of supreme sadness.
Help me to rise each day
And carry on, even though my heart is broken.
Give me the strength to someday move past
This dark place, and point me toward
The place where you most want me to be.
Through Christ our Lord.
Amen.

Watch, O Lord

Watch, O Lord, with those who wake,
or watch, or weep tonight,
and give your angels and saints
charge over those who sleep.

Tend your sick ones, O Lord Christ,
rest your weary ones,
bless your dying ones,
soothe your suffering ones,
pity your afflicted ones
shield your joyous ones.

And all for your love's sake.

St. Augustine

Chapter Nine

Other Options: Adoption

He chose us in Christ before the foundation of the world to be holy and blameless before him in love. He destined us for adoption as his children through Jesus Christ according to the good pleasure of his will, to the praise of his glorious grace that he freely bestowed on us in the Beloved.

Ephesians 1:4-6

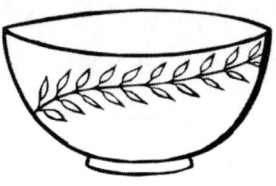

BEFORE MY HUSBAND AND I MARRIED, we attended a marriage-preparation class, which is a requirement in many Christian churches. We talked about the issues most likely to cause conflict in a marriage, such as money and in-laws. And while we talked about children, we never discussed what we might do if we had trouble conceiving. It's too bad, because an estimated 15 percent of couples will have trouble conceiving. Discussing their options early might save them from disappointing surprises later on.

Since the marriage-prep classes don't cover the subject, it's a good idea for couples who are trying to conceive to begin talking about what will happen if their attempts fail. Whether we are just beginning to pursue treatment or we're farther along in the process, it helps to know what the options are. Even within a strong marriage people are often surprised to learn, for instance, that their spouses are deeply uncomfortable with the idea of adoption, or that they wouldn't mind a life without children.

For couples who choose not to pursue fertility treatments, or for those whose treatments don't succeed, there are two primary options: adoption and living childfree. Ending the pursuit of biological parenthood can be a wrenching time, but both adoption and childfree living can be wonderful options, full of excitement and deep satisfaction. The challenge is deciding which one to follow.

Considering Adoption

Perusing the Bible, it seems clear that God is a fan of adoption. There is Moses, of course, and Esther in the Old Testament. More importantly for Christians, there is Jesus, whom Joseph loved and cared for even though they had no biological ties. And, as Paul states again and again throughout his epistles, our relationship to God is one of adopted children to our adoptive father. Although Jesus was God's only begotten son, we are God's children too, whom God loves unconditionally.

And yet, adoption is not for everyone—not even for every Christian. Even though my daughter joined our family by adoption, an experience that was in every way as wonderful and awe-inspiring as giving birth, I recognize that not everyone is comfortable with the idea of raising a child they did not conceive. And people who are profoundly uncomfortable with the idea, even if they want to favor it, should not adopt. But there are also many people who are open to the idea of adoption but still harbor reservations. So how does a couple decide if adoption is right for them?

Research and prayer are two excellent places to start. Research—reading books, attending seminars, and talking to adoptive parents—will answer the many questions that arise when someone is considering adoption. It can resolve some of the most obvious fears and raise issues that are rarely considered, all the while guiding couples toward a carefully considered decision.

The other essential component to making a decision on adoption is prayer. This is a huge decision that mustn't be rushed or taken lightly. To determine what is truly in our hearts takes time and quiet prayer. Listening to God in prayer may not change the mind of anyone set against adopting; but for those who are open to the idea, committed prayer can guide them in ways that books and seminars sometimes can't.

The Process of Adopting

Those of us who want to adopt have many decisions to make. Do we want to adopt domestically or internationally? Will it be an open adoption, in which we continue some level of contact with the birth parents? Are we set on an infant, or will we consider a toddler or an older child? Will we go with a private agency or public? Would we accept a foster child who might later be available for adoption?

No matter what kind of adoption, everyone must complete a home study in which a social worker interviews everyone in the family, visits the home, and makes certain the parents are prepared and fit for adoptive parenting. Once the home study is complete, the family waits for the referral of a child. This can take weeks, months or years, depending on the type of adoption. Once the child is placed in the adoptive home, there is a waiting period that includes additional visits from a social worker to ensure the adoption is proceeding smoothly. The family then goes to court to finalize the adoption.

Many people who are considering adoption are put off by the process of adopting. Sometimes they have witnessed the mountains of paperwork and the months of uncertainty that adoptive parents have faced. They have heard how social workers come to the home of families wanting to adopt and ask all sorts of nosy questions. A few might know a couple who took custody of an infant only to have the birth parents change their minds. It might seem like it's just not worth the hassle, especially if they've endured years of trying to conceive.

Cooperating with the home study is a way of guaranteeing that the process works for everyone.

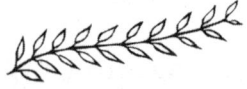

I'm not saying the paperwork and social-worker visits are fun, but they certainly are necessary. The child's safety and well-being are paramount and require agencies and social workers to examine would-be adoptive parents carefully. Would any of us want an agency placing a child in a home without examining the family first? Cooperating with the home study is a way of guaranteeing that the process works for everyone.

I like to compare it to the marriage preparation courses my church required engaged couples to attend. I felt that I didn't need a class to tell me that my husband and I were ready to be married, but if the mandatory class helped other couples who weren't ready to realize it, then the weekend we spent at it wasn't wasted. So it is with the adoption process: If everyone goes through the same set of interviews and paperwork, both adoption professionals and families can determine whether we are ready for this momentous change in our lives.

In our case, I actually found the process to be less cumbersome than I'd anticipated. Perhaps because I'd read horror stories about how difficult the home study was, I was pleasantly surprised when it finally came time to complete it. We were able to pull all our documents together, complete the questions, and conduct our interviews in under two months. It was a bit inconvenient and time-consuming, but the end result—the arrival of our daughter a few months later—was worth every moment.

Common Concerns about Adopting

I'm not an expert on adoption, but I have talked to enough people to know that there are concerns about adoption and the process of adopting that tend to come up again and again. The following answers may not resolve any concerns with finality, but they may provide a launching pad for further discussion, research and prayer, and add the perspective of someone whose adventures in adoption turned out happily.

Can I love an adopted child as much as I'd love a biological child?

I usually answer this by pointing out that we love our spouses deeply even though we share no biological bond with them. And most parents, when asked what we love most about being a parent, won't mention our genetic link to our children. Instead, we talk about the thrill of watching a little one's personality unfold, or the challenge of guiding a child to live responsibly and morally, or the unconditional love and deep pride we feel as we watch our children find their place in the world. These feelings have nothing to do with whether a child is adopted or not; they have everything to do with the bond parents forge with our children through years of shared experiences.

Parents with more than one child also say that while we love each child with equal intensity, we also love them differently because each child is such a different person. In my experience, love—for a child or a spouse—is not a thunderbolt that strikes all at once. It builds gradually, through shared moments and experiences, until one day we realize we would do anything to protect the object of our love.

What if there's something wrong with the child I adopt? How do I know what I'm getting into?

There are no guarantees that the child you adopt will be problem-free. But then, there's no guarantee that any child you give birth to will be problem-free either. Parenthood is full of risks. We try to minimize them, but we never eliminate them. Every day, uncomplicated pregnancies end in unexplained stillbirth; children fall ill; some die; and we can't always prevent it. Love requires emotional risk, but the risk is miniscule compared to the benefits.

It's true that adopted children are slightly more likely to seek out counseling than their non-adopted counterparts, especially in adolescence when most people struggle to forge their identities. But the differences are very small and largely eliminated when the adopted child reaches adulthood. In actuality, the number of difficult adoptions is very low.

Additionally, we live in a time when it is perhaps easier than ever to be adopted. Adoption was once considered something of a secret. Many adoptees never knew the circumstances of their birth...or found out by accident. Now there are adoption support groups, online services that connect adoptees to one another, and a wide range of other resources available to families through adoption agencies or in their communities. Adoptive families now routinely celebrate the way they were formed instead of being secretive about it.

What if the birth parents change their mind and take their child back?

The cases in which birth parents change their minds and regain custody are wrenching. They are also very rare. Most adoptions, whether domestic or international, try to ensure that the birth parents that make an adoption plan are given some flexibility in their decision. Sometimes the birth of a baby prompts uncertainty in people who thought their decisions were certain. Parenthood comes with its own risks, and the first days after a child's birth are a risky and vulnerable time for adoptive parents. While it's certainly difficult when an adoption falls through in its first few days, it's better that it happen then rather than months or even years later when lengthy, draining court fights are possible.

For couples who are extremely nervous about the role of birth parents in an adoption, there are several options. Children from other countries are generally made available for adoption only after their birth parents have ended their rights to the children. It is extremely rare for an international adoption to be affected by a birth parent's change of heart. Toddlers and older children in the U.S. are also usually available for adoption only after the birth parents' rights have ended. Talking with a social worker may help illuminate the risks and recommend ways to lessen them.

I want to adopt, but my spouse is against it.
This is a difficult situation for which there are no easy solutions. In talking this over with our spouses, it's important not only to share our opinions but also the strength of our feelings. Is the partner who opposes adoption lukewarm or adamant in his or her opposition? For the spouse who wants to adopt, are there other options that he or she is willing to consider?

If both partners are firmly entrenched in their opinions, it's probably best to involve a neutral third party such as a pastor or therapist. With the help of someone outside the marriage, it might be easier to view the situation from our spouse's perspective.

I know that there are many children out there who need homes, but I don't know if I'm patient or generous enough to adopt.

Adoption is not charity work. Couples who adopt are not saving the child from an uncertain future; they are simply expanding their family. It's unfair for a child to be adopted by people who see themselves as his or her savior instead of merely the child's parents. Adoptive parenting doesn't require any more patience or generosity than biological parenting. Are any of us patient and generous enough to be parents? Maybe not, but that shouldn't prevent us from trying.

Why does adoption cost so much? It's unfair that some families want to adopt but can't afford it.

It's true that adoption can be fairly expensive, depending on the type of adoption. But adoption is time- and labor-intensive work that requires the efforts of many people to succeed, and it takes money to carry out the duties of social workers, foster caregivers, translators, administrators, and others.

The price of resolving infertility, whether it's for medical treatment or adoption, is one of the biggest injustices of the entire ordeal. Having said that, there are ways to lower the costs associated with adoption. In general, domestic adoptions cost less than international adoptions, and adoptions through public agencies cost less than those through private agencies. Many companies offer their employees adoption assistance, and there are state and federal tax credits available to families who adopt. And one nice thing about the fees for adoption is that they usually guarantee you a child, unlike medical treatment, which offers only the chance of a child.

Whenever someone is contemplating adoption, these concerns and others loom large. But it's a disservice not to talk about the joys as well. In the midst of these and other concerns, we sometimes forget to talk about how much joy there is in adoption. The sense of accomplishment that comes from completing the study; the anxious wait for a referral; the thrill of seeing a picture of our child for the first time; the moment we hold our child for the first time; and the milestones that follow, from first words to first day of school, with all of the attendant pride and awe that comes with being someone's parent. It's important not to let common concerns blind us to the miracle of adoption.

At the same time we have to be honest with ourselves about whether we're ready for this enormous step, even if it is the only option we have to become parents. It is normal to have some doubts, but we must have the courage to proceed slowly or not at all if our own particular doubts are telling us to do so. Every child deserves to have a family that is over-the-moon ecstatic about the prospect of his or her arrival. A careful process of discernment should reveal whether adoption is the right step, and whether that excitement is living in our hearts.

PRAYER AND REFLECTION

Isaiah 43:5-6
Do not fear, for I am with you;
I will bring your offspring from the east
    and from the west I will gather you.
I will say to the north, "Give them up!" and to the south,
    "Do not withhold; bring my sons from far away
    and my daughters from the end of the earth."

Romans 8:14-23
For all who are led by the Spirit of God are children of
God. For you did not receive a spirit of slavery to fall
back into fear, but you received a spirit of adoption.
When we cry, "Abba, Father!" it is that very Spirit bearing
witness with our spirit that we are children of God, and
if children, then heirs, heirs of God and joint heirs with
Christ—if, in fact, we suffer with him so that we may
also be glorified with him. I consider that the sufferings
of this present time are not worth comparing with the
glory about to be revealed to us.

For the creation awaits with eager longing for the
revealing of the children of God; for the creation was
subjected to futility, not of its own will but by the will
of the one who subjected it, in hope that the creation
itself will be set free from its bondage to decay and will

obtain the freedom of the glory of the children of God. We know that the whole creation has been groaning in labor pains until now; and not only the creation, but we ourselves, who have the first fruits of the Spirit, groan inwardly while we wait for adoption, the redemption of our bodies.

Adoption Prayer
Occasional Services,
A Companion to the Lutheran Book of Worship

Father of the fatherless, you give your children a home in which to dwell; and like a loving mother you gather us into your household. We give you thanks for the child who has come to bless this family and for the parents who have taken this child to be their own. By the power of your Holy Spirit, fill [name(s) of parent or parents] with trust, understanding and affection; and, through this child in our midst, enable us better to know the mystery that we are all your children by adoption; through Jesus Christ our Lord.

A Prayer for Discernment

Please God,

Help me to know what to do.

Will you send me one of your children through adoption?

Is this how our family is meant to grow?

I know it's not an easy thing to decide.

The path to it can seem lonely and difficult.

You know, O Lord, whether this is the right thing for us.

Help us to know too.

Amen.

Chapter Ten

Other Options: A Family of Two

"Do not let your hearts be troubled.
Believe in God; believe also in me."

John 14:1

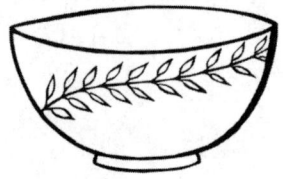

PARENTHOOD IS A REWARDING and deeply-satisfying role. It is also perhaps the most difficult and time-consuming work of many people's lives. There is no way to prepare for how much energy it takes. No matter how much parents want to maintain the relationships and interests we had before children, we inevitably must make sacrifices to accommodate the duties of parenthood.

A generation ago it was expected that a couple who married young enough to have children would do so, but no longer. Increasingly, married couples are deciding that the sacrifices required by children are too great, deciding instead to devote their lives to their work, their passions and relationships, and especially their marriage. These couples—many of whom have not encountered infertility—lead meaningful lives filled with friends, family, careers, hobbies and volunteer work. Some people who have made a conscious decision not to have children prefer to be called "childfree" rather than "childless," to emphasize the positive aspects of life without children rather than stressing what they don't have.

When a couple has tried without success to become parents, imagining life without children can feel like an enormous disappointment. There is no easy way to dismiss these dreams of having a family; the only way to move past them is to grieve for the loss they represent. But many people who have planned on having children never considered the benefits of living childfree. Perhaps by examining the benefits, and by praying for guidance and actively imagining themselves as childfree, a couple can decide if this path is right for them.

The Gift of Time

Ask a childfree couple what they most enjoy about their life and they will probably first mention everything they are able to do: sleep late, travel extensively, eat out frequently, and enjoy one another's company without the demands of children. But while leisurely meals and late mornings sound wonderful, they might also seem empty or selfish to anyone who longs for a meaningful life. Most of us want to do more with ourselves than simply pursue pleasure.

Living without children, though, is much more than leisurely meals and late mornings. What a couple gains when they decide not to have children is time — time they would have spent changing diapers, carpooling, packing lunches, and standing at soccer games. The question for this couple becomes: What do we do with our time now? It's a question parents should ask themselves as well, but rarely do. Many parents would like to write a book, or travel to Africa, or start their own business, but we think, I can't do that and raise children at the same time. And so our dreams are placed on a shelf, hidden behind the demands of childrearing.

When a couple decides not to have children, they must do the hard work of deciding what it is they want to do. Some decide they want to invest their time in their careers. Perhaps they have careers that they love already and want to continue in their chosen field. For others, the decision to live childfree might prompt a career change to something perhaps more demanding but ultimately more satisfying.

Others may decide to invest their time in volunteer work as a way to find meaning and make the world a better place. There's certainly no shortage of people and organizations who need the time and talents of others to succeed. Living without children also frees up time to spend on interests and hobbies, from community theatre to marathon running to collecting antiques. And perhaps most importantly, the childfree can afford to invest more time and energy into being a better spouse, friend, sibling, aunt or uncle. It is not easy for the childfree to decide what to invest their time and resources in, but the payoff is living a life they've chosen rather than merely stumbled into.

Connecting with Others

Many of us have had close friendships that change when our friends become parents. Gradually or all at once, they are less available to meet for coffee or a round of golf, and when we do see them it's difficult to converse without interruptions. Once their children reach school age, it seems as though all their free time is spent at baseball practices and ballet recitals, and our friendships suffer another blow. It is possible to maintain friendships between parents and non-parents, but it also takes a great deal of time and commitment.

However, the childfree often enjoy deeply-satisfying

friendships based on shared interests and the freedom to enjoy them. I know childfree women who walk together daily and are able to exercise as they share long conversations; they often stop for coffee or head out to dinner together afterward, and they are able to do so because they have fewer demands on their time. I also know men who are able to get away for fishing and golf trips more frequently than their friends who have children. The time they spend with their friends is clearly cherished, and it buoys their spirits long after their travels are over. Obviously parents can go on walks or fishing trips as well, but the demands of raising children inevitably crowd out some leisure time and time spent maintaining relationships.

It's useful to think about why we want to be parents, to see if we can find other ways to fulfill those desires.

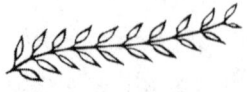

It's useful to think about why we want to be parents, to see if we can find other ways to fulfill those desires. The childfree are often able—and sometimes especially well-suited—to care for ailing neighbors or elderly parents. Caring for the ill and elderly is a great need in our society, especially as people live longer than previous generations did, and there is wisdom to be gleaned from older people and satisfaction in meeting their needs.

Those who want to spend time around children likely have nieces and nephews or the children of friends to spoil. I was fortunate enough to have an aunt who did not have children, and some of my most wonderful childhood memories were of riding the elevator in her glamorous apartment building and dressing up to go to the theatre with her. There are also roles as mentors, coaches and teachers that can satisfy a need to teach and encourage the young.

Finally, childfree couples are able to spend time enriching their marriages and loving their spouses. Again, that's not to say that parents don't enjoy wonderful relationships, but couples without children can make their marriage an absolute priority and are able to do activities—such as retreats or extended volunteer work— that strengthen their bond without worrying about other responsibilities. They are free, within the context of a Christian marriage and their relationship with God, to be devoted to one another.

Creating a Legacy

Parents often speak of their children as their legacy— that no matter what else we do in life, if we are able to raise children successfully, we will have left our mark on the world. Especially as Christians, we are concerned with our legacy and our duty to help bring about God's kingdom on Earth. It's a natural impulse, even for those who don't believe in God, to leave something of themselves alive in their children after they die. This leads many of us to want to become parents in the first place, and what makes a childfree life less attractive to some.

But there are limitless ways to create a legacy

outside of raising children. There is medical research that uncovers cures to terrible diseases, and music that lifts the soul of those who hear it, and orphanages in developing countries that give clothing, food and hope to children who might otherwise have none. There is the neighbor who always shows up with a casserole when someone has died, and the co-worker who treats everyone in the office with dignity and respect, and the swimming coach whose kindness and expectations encourage everyone to do their best.

We all have the capacity to leave a legacy, whether it includes children or not. In fact, as sons and daughters of God, we have a responsibility not to waste the gifts God has given us. It is up to us to decide whether that legacy will include raising children or not, but no matter what we decide, we can—we must—still work to make our world a better place.

PRAYER AND REFLECTION

Isaiah 30:20-21
Though the Lord may give you the bread of adversity and the water of affliction, yet your teacher will not hide himself any more, but your eyes shall see your teacher. And when you turn to the right or when you turn to the left, your ears shall hear a word behind you, saying, "This is the way; walk in it."

Proverbs 2:6-9
For the Lord gives wisdom; from his mouth come knowledge and understanding; he stores up sound wisdom for the upright; he is a shield to those who walk blamelessly, guarding the paths of justice and preserving the way of his faithful ones. Then you will understand righteousness and justice and equity, every good path.

Prayer for Discernment

Dear Lord,
This wasn't the life we had in mind.
We wanted to raise children in our home,
To teach them about your love
And enjoy them in our old age.

And yet, we realize there is much work
That needs to be done outside of raising children of our own.
There are your sick ones to care for,
And your sorrowful ones to console.
Are you asking that we follow a different path?
Help us to know, dear God, what to do,
And help us to love the life you've prepared for us.
We ask this in Jesus' name.
Amen.

Look upon Us, O Lord

Look upon us, O Lord,
and let all the darkness of our souls
vanish before the beams of thy brightness.
Fill us with holy love,
and open to us the treasures of thy wisdom.
All our desire is known unto thee,
therefore perfect what thou hast begun,
and what thy Spirit has awakened us to ask in prayer.
We seek thy face,
turn thy face unto us and show us thy glory.
Then shall our longing be satisfied,
and our peace shall be perfect.

St. Augustine

Chapter Eleven

Waiting in Hope

For surely I know the plans I have for you, says the Lord,
plans for your welfare and not for harm,
to give you a future with hope.

Jeremiah 29:11

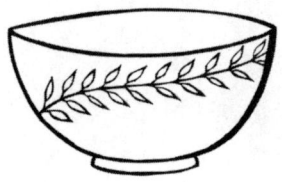

ADVENT IS MY FAVORITE TIME OF YEAR. I used to become overwhelmed by the demands of Christmas, frantically rushing around, buying presents, and making cookies out of a sense of obligation rather than joy. But after thinking and praying about it, I decided to emphasize Advent in the weeks before Christmas and to protect the religious season from the commercial demands that surround it. I began to light an Advent wreath, and the mere act of lighting a candle every night seemed to slow down time and make me cherish it much more.

Advent celebrates a pregnancy, which makes it a strange example of how we should face our infertility. But consider again how Mary must have felt about her pregnancy: confused, frightened and overwhelmed with this strange and unexpected news. Even with God's direct intervention—even with a visit from the angel Gabriel—Mary is troubled at first by this turn of events.

And yet, after prayer and reflection, Mary tells God, "Let it be with me according to your word" (Luke 1:38). She manages, after the initial shock, to wait with hope for the birth of Jesus. She could have raged against God for doing this to her; she could have withdrawn, or run away, or cursed her fate. But she listened to her heart and accepted God's plan, and in doing so she turned an unplanned pregnancy into a "yes" that would save the world.

For most of us, our infertility is unexpected and unwelcome. We're probably not ready at first to accept this change in the plans we have for our life; we may need time to withdraw, or rage against God, or curse the injustice of it all. We can't reach a place of hope until we've had a chance to address our suffering. This suffering, as painful as it is, helps us to grow spiritually, connects us with others who suffer, and helps us to understand Jesus and our faith better.

But after much reflection, and perhaps some anger and fear, we may be ready to listen to our hearts and say "yes" to what God has in store for us. We can choose contentment and joy. We can be happy with what we have no matter what our future holds. It takes strength and determination to wait with hope for God's plan to unfold, but God has given each of us what we need to be strong, determined people.

Growth through Suffering

When my husband and I were in the midst of suffering from infertility, I had two primary spiritual reactions: I prayed for my pain to go away, and I wanted to know why we had to suffer so. For a long time I tried to find the exact lesson I believed God was trying to teach me through our infertility. At one point I decided we were suffering so I could learn patience. It seemed like a very smart move on God's part: Teach me patience by denying me something I really wanted. I had to give God credit for that one.

And so I tried to practice patience. I even got pretty good at it. I began to think, Okay God, I've learned my lesson. You can give us a baby now. Still nothing. And as the months progressed I became angry and deflated. I despaired of ever figuring out what God was trying to teach us.

Who doesn't try to avoid suffering when we feel it bearing down on us? And who, in the midst of a suffering such as infertility, doesn't wonder, Why is this happening to me? It is a natural reaction when we find ourselves enduring great pain. Even Jesus pleaded and questioned as his death drew near. Standing in the garden of Gethsemane the night before his crucifixion, he pleads with God to take this cup, this pain, away: "Abba, Father, for you all things are possible; remove this cup from me; yet not what I want but what you want" (Mark 14:36). And the next day, as he is dying on the cross he asks, "My God, my God, why have you forsaken me?" (Mark 15:34). If Jesus voiced these thoughts while he suffered, how can we hope to escape the same questions and struggles?

In my own case, I gradually began to search not for the one lesson God was trying to teach me, but for the many lessons I could learn with what I'd been given. And when I started looking, the lessons were everywhere. I had indeed learned to be more patient, and that was a blessing whether I was to have children or not. I had learned so much about infertility that I was able to help several friends, and friends of friends, who were just beginning to navigate the worlds of assisted reproduction and adoption. These lessons may or may not be what God had in mind for me to learn, but I have a feeling God was pleased with my efforts anyway.

Accepting the Cross

When I was growing up, whenever I encountered a difficulty, my mother would advise me to "offer it up for the poor souls in purgatory." It never made sense to me: How could my troubles help someone else, whether they were in purgatory or not? Could we really transfer our pain to assist another person?

I've come to understand this a bit differently after my struggle to have children. As a result of infertility, I found myself with greater empathy for people in pain everywhere. I tried to become more generous with my time and resources because I had a glimmer of what it was to truly suffer, and I wanted to help ease the pain of others, whether they were neighbors suffering from cancer or tsunami victims in Indonesia. I felt, deep in my heart, a kinship with people all over the world that I'd never met, simply because they'd suffered something incomprehensible. I pondered how this sense of shared pain often moves us to act, and how we find redemption and meaning in our suffering when we can help others in their time of need. We each have the ability to be the face of God to people in pain, and often an ordeal of our own is the impetus we need to act.

Deep suffering brings us closer to Jesus as well, because we begin to understand the awesome sacrifice he made for us when he died on the cross. We suffer usually because we have no other choice; Jesus suffered because he agreed to die for our sins. By contemplating this mystery, we come closer to understanding how, after his questioning, he was able to say, "Yet not what I want, but what you want" (Mark 14:36). This is the spiritual growth and maturity that suffering can bring.

It also helps to look at how Jesus confronted the mystery of suffering. He did not try to explain why accidents happen, why people get sick, why death and disease strike with such regularity. What Jesus did was try to relieve that suffering whenever and however he could. Jesus never advised the people he met to give in to suffering; he always urged them to fight to become better and more whole. But he also showed us that suffering and sickness can bring blessings we could never imagine. They teach us that life is precious, that we should reach out to others, that we can call on

Jesus always urged people to fight to become better and more whole.

God's help, and that above all, we should trust in God's goodness, even when God's plan is hidden from our view.

Finding Joy

We think, when we start trying to conceive a child, that this child will bring us happiness.

So often we equate joy with getting what we want. But think, for a moment, about the joyful mysteries of the Catholic Rosary: the angel Gabriel announcing to Mary that she will have a son; Mary visiting her cousin Elizabeth, who will give birth to John the Baptist even though she had despaired of conceiving; the birth of Jesus; his presentation in the temple; and the finding of the child Jesus in the temple after he was lost.

They are events filled with surprise and often trepidation. Mary certainly didn't ask to become pregnant before marriage; Elizabeth had given up on ever having a child because of her advanced age; and Mary and Joseph were filled with fear and anxiety before they found Jesus. Their joy—and ours too—comes not in getting what we want, but in accepting God's will and finding the good in it, even when we don't understand it.

I don't mean that we should try to convince ourselves that we don't really want a baby, when it's clearly our deepest desire. We shouldn't try to deny the pain we're feeling. But with or without a child, our lives are full of blessings and grace. We have everything we need to find contentment, even joy, whether our wishes are fulfilled or not.

Once I started looking for blessings in the midst of our infertility, I found them everywhere. There was the blessing of a resilient marriage that grew even stronger after it was tested by infertility. There were friends and family whose care pulled us out of many difficult days. There were nurses whose care and compassion never failed, even when they were forced to call with disappointing news.

And after our son was born and our daughter was adopted, I found it a blessing that it had taken us so long to have children, because I was so very pleased with the family we ended up with. I don't believe they are the only children we could have had, or the exact two that were meant for us, but I wouldn't want our struggle to have turned out any other way.

In one of her best-loved poems, Emily Dickinson wrote, "Hope is the thing with feathers—/That perches in the soul—/And sings the tune without the words/And never stops—at all—." So how do we remain hopeful in the face of uncertainty, when the clear plans we've made for our lives are battered by disappointments and pain? We remember that hope is not blind optimism, nor arrogant certainty, nor wishful thinking. Rather, it is the knowledge that God is always with us, and that we will endure hard times to see a better day. None of us knows what our future holds, whether it's the family we'd always dreamed of or something entirely unimagined at this point. We know only that God is good, and that God's goodness will prevail in the end. That is why we wait, not in fear, but in hope.

PRAYER AND REFLECTION

Lamentations 3:17-18; 21-24

My soul is bereft of peace; I have forgotten what happiness is; so I say, "Gone is my glory, and all that I had hoped for from the Lord."

But this I call to mind, and therefore I have hope: The steadfast love of the Lord never ceases, his mercies never come to an end; they are new every morning; great is your faithfulness. "The Lord is my portion," says my soul, "therefore I will hope in him."

2 Corinthians 1:3-7

Blessed be the God and Father of our Lord Jesus Christ, the Father of mercies and the God of all consolation, who consoles us in all our affliction, so that we may be able to console those who are in any affliction with the consolation with which we ourselves are consoled by God. For just as the sufferings of Christ are abundant for us, so also our consolation is abundant for us, so also our consolation is abundant through Christ.

Prayer of Thanksgiving

Dear God,
I thank you for my life,
For the chance to enjoy your creation
And to love the people around me.
Sometimes I forget what a glorious thing it is
To be alive.
Thank you also for the suffering you send,
For the opportunity to grow in faith,
To understand a glimmer of what Jesus endured,
And to learn what it means to be fully human.
Help me to remember that everything unfolds
According to your plan.
Please keep hope alive in my heart,
And help me to act with the strength and knowledge
That suffering has taught me.
We ask this in Jesus' name.
Amen.

Give Us Grace

Lord God, whose blessed Son our Savior gave his body to be whipped and his face to be spit upon: Give us grace to accept joyfully the sufferings of the present time, confident of the glory that shall be revealed; through Jesus Christ our Lord.

The Book of Common Prayer 1979

Infertility Resources

Fertile Thoughts (www.fertilethoughts.com)
Online forums on the medical and emotional aspects of infertility treatment, adoption, surrogacy, donor gametes and other issues.

Hannah's Prayer Ministries (www.hannah.org)
An online Christian support network for those suffering from infertility, pregnancy loss, adoption loss, and early infant death.

The International Council on Infertility Information Dissemination, Inc. (www.inciid.org)
One of the oldest and largest online communities for infertility, adoption and childfree living, with answers from experts and peer support forums.

RESOLVE (www.resolve.org)
The National Infertility Association. RESOLVE offers local support groups, online forums, and national advocacy on issues like insurance coverage for medical treatment of infertility.

Saint Gerard.com (www.saintgerard.com)
A prayer list and support message boards devoted to St. Gerard Majella, an eighteenth-century Catholic saint popularly known as a patron of the infertile and mothers.

Shaohannah's Hope (www.shaohannahshope.org)
A ministry founded by musician Steven Curtis Chapman to care for orphans and reduce the cost of adoption for Christian families.

Stepping Stones (www.bethany.org/step)
A ministry of Bethany Christian Services, Stepping Stones provides local support groups, a bi-monthly newsletter, and online forums and resources about infertility.

References

American Cancer Society. "What are the Risk Factors for Ovarian Cancer?" (www.cancer.org).

American College of Obstetricians and Gynecologists. "Multiple Pregnancies and Birth: Considering Fertility Treatments" (www.acog.org).

American Society for Reproductive Medicine (www.asrm.org).

Aronson, Diane and Levert, Suzanne. *Resolving Infertility* (Collins Living, 2001).

Centers for Disease Control and Prevention (www.cdc.gov).

Johnston, Patricia Irwin. *Adopting After Infertility* (Perspectives Press, 1994).

MedlinePlus Infertility (www.nlm.nih.gov/medlineplus/infertility.html).

National Institute of Child Health and Human Services, "Research on Miscarriage and Stillbirth" (www.nichd.nih.gov).

Sher, Geoffrey. *Fertility and Conception: A Complete Guide to Getting Pregnant* (DK Adult, 2003).

Silber, Sherman J. *How to Get Pregnant* (Little, Brown and Company, 2007).

Weschler, Toni. *Taking Charge of Your Fertility: The Definitive Guide to Natural Birth Control, Pregnancy Achievement, and Reproductive Health* (Collins Living, 2006).